ANTI-INFLAMMATORY DIET COOKBOOK FOR BEGINNERS (FULL COLOR EDITION)

Lots of Easy, Quick and Delicious Recipes to reduce Inflammation and Improve your Health. 28-Day Meal Plan and Weekly Shopping List

Emily Lawrenson

INTRODUCTION

The Anti-Inflammatory Diet, as the name suggests, consists of reducing inflammation in the body. This diet is based on the idea that the foods we eat can have a powerful effect on our health and that eating certain foods helps to reduce inflammation. The anti-inflammatory diet is based on the concept of consuming a diet rich in fruits, vegetables, fish, and whole grains, while avoiding foods that may increase inflammation, such as processed foods, refined sugar, and saturated fats. This diet has been gaining a lot of popularity in recent years, due to the health benefits it provides. As proven by many studies, the diet reduces the risk of chronic diseases and also improves heart health. Moreover, the Anti-Inflammatory Diet has been linked to improved mental health, as well as better sleep quality and energy levels. The main foods of the diet are those rich in antioxidants, vitamins, and minerals, and low in saturated fats and refined sugar. Among the main ones are: fruits and vegetables, whole grains, nuts and seeds, fish and lean proteins, and healthy fats. Regular physical exercise can also help reduce inflammation, as well as improve health and overall wellbeing. By following the diet and its guidelines, it is therefore possible to improve overall health and consequently reduce the risk of developing chronic diseases.

THE BENEFITS OF THE ANTI-INFLAMMATORY DIET

The anti-inflammatory diet is quickly becoming one of the most popular diets among Americans. This diet focuses on reducing inflammation in the body, which can help reduce the risk of chronic diseases such as heart disease, diabetes, and certain types of cancer. The diet emphasizes how important it is to consume a variety of whole, naturally anti-inflammatory foods, reducing or eliminating processed foods and refined sugars altogether. Fruits and vegetables are rich in essential vitamins and minerals as well as powerful antioxidants that can help reduce inflammation. Eating a good amount of fruits and vegetables of various colors ensures that you get a wide range of essential nutrients. In addition to the beneficial nutrients found in fruits and vegetables, the anti-inflammatory diet also encourages the consumption of healthy proteins, such as lean meats, fish, eggs, and legumes. Protein is essential for cell and tissue growth and repair, and also helps provide energy and regulate metabolism. Lastly, the anti-inflammatory diet encourages the consumption of healthy carbohydrates like whole grains, starchy vegetables, and legumes. These foods are high in fiber, which helps keep you feeling full and helps facilitate digestion. They also provide slow-burning energy to keep you energized throughout the day. Moreover, the diet helps promote weight loss and provide essential nutrients to keep you healthy and energized.

FOODS TO EAT

Now let's come to the main foods of the anti-inflammatory diet: Fruit: Fruit is rich in antioxidants, which can help reduce inflammation in the body. Berries, cherries, apples, citrus fruits and pomegranates are all great sources of antioxidants. Vegetables: Vegetables are an excellent source of vitamins, minerals and fibre, all of which are important for reducing inflammation. Leafy green vegetables, cruciferous vegetables and colourful vegetables are particularly beneficial. Legumes: Legumes such as beans, lentils and chickpeas are another great source of fibre and plant-based proteins; legumes are also rich in phytonutrients. Nuts and seeds: Nuts and seeds are rich in healthy fats, fibre and antioxidants. Almonds, walnuts, flax seeds and chia seeds are some of the best options for an anti-inflammatory diet. Fish and seafood: Fish and seafood are excellent sources of omega-3 fatty acids. Wild salmon, sardines, mackerel and shellfish such as oysters, mussels and clams are all highly recommended. Whole grains: Whole grains are rich in fibre, B vitamins and antioxidants. Choose whole grains such as quinoa, buckwheat and oats. Herbs and spices: turmeric, ginger and chilli are the most recommended, being excellent sources of antioxidants. Healthy fats: Healthy fats such as extra virgin olive oil, avocado and coconut oil are all great sources of anti-inflammatory fats. Eggs: they are also an excellent source of protein and healthy fats, which can help reduce inflammation in the body. Finally, something very important in addition to a healthy diet is to stay hydrated by drinking plenty of water during the day.

FOODS TO AVOID

As we have already pointed out before, now we will list what foods to avoid, since they are high in sugars and processed fats, such as fried foods, processed meats and sugary snacks. Processed meats such as wurstel, bacon and sausages are rich in saturated fats and nitrates. Undoubtedly they increase inflammation in the body as well as being linked to a higher risk of heart disease, cancer and other health problems. Fried foods such as french fries, onion rings, mozzarella sticks etc. are rich in unhealthy fats. Refined carbohydrates such as white bread, white rice and sugary snacks are rich in simple sugars and can raise blood sugar levels. Processed foods such as ready-made and canned foods are often high in sodium, preservatives and other unhealthy additives. Alcoholic beverages such as beer, wine and spirits are to be avoided if following an anti-inflammatory diet, as it is known that alcohol can be lethal to inflammation. Sugary drinks such as sodas, energy drinks and sweetened teas are high in calories and can raise blood sugar levels.

In general, following an anti-inflammatory diet means avoiding foods high in fats, processed and high in sugars, as well as processed meats, fried foods, refined carbohydrates, processed and canned foods, alcoholic beverages and sugary drinks.

EATING OUT AND SHOPPING TIPS

Eating out is one of life's great pleasures, so if you're following a diet like this, it will definitely be a challenge for you to stick to it. However, with the right strategies, you can enjoy a meal at a restaurant without compromising your diet. When eating out, start by doing some research in advance: for example, before choosing the restaurant, check the online menu and make sure there are dishes that meet your dietary requirements. If you have been invited to a dinner and you couldn't refuse, ask the waiter if the chef can accommodate your needs, explaining your situation. Most restaurants are willing to make changes to meals, such as using olive oil instead of butter or leaving out certain ingredients. It is also important to check portion sizes when eating out. Ask the waiter to bring you a smaller portion or to put half of your meal aside to take home. This will help you avoid overeating. When grocery shopping, always be sure to read labels. Look for foods that are free of preservatives and additives. Choose fresh, unprocessed foods as well as seasonal fruits and vegetables if possible. When buying canned foods, look for products with fewer ingredients. Avoid foods that contain added sugars, artificial sweeteners and fats. Choose organic, non-GMO products if possible. If you are buying frozen foods, choose products that are low in sodium, sugar and saturated fats. Look for products "all natural" or "organic". Finally, don't forget to stock your pantry with healthy snacks. Following an anti-inflammatory diet doesn't have to be difficult; with the right strategies, you can enjoy delicious dishes both at home and in restaurants. By reading labels, choosing fresh, unprocessed foods and checking portion sizes, you can stick to your diet and still enjoy a variety of flavors.

COOKING TECHNIQUES FOR ANTI-INFLAMMATORY FOODS

Now we will list the best cooking techniques when following an anti-inflammatory diet. The most well-known and important technique is without a doubt STEAM COOKING: this cooking method allows to preserve the important vitamins, minerals and other nutrients present in the food.
BAKING: it is a great way to cook meat and fish, as it helps to seal in the moisture and prevent the food from drying out.
Baking also helps to retain the flavor of the food.
STIR-FRY: it is another important cooking technique for the anti-inflammatory diet. This cooking method helps to retain the flavor and important nutrients and other compounds present in the food.
BOILING: it is an important cooking technique for the anti-inflammatory diet. Boiling helps to preserve the important vitamins and minerals present in the foods, as well as other important compounds. It also helps to make the food easier to digest and helps to prevent the food from becoming overcooked.

GRILLING: it may sound strange, but (although not too often) grilling foods such as meat or fish is allowed too.

SLOW COOKING: it is another important cooking technique for the anti-inflammatory diet. As with steam cooking, this method helps to preserve the important vitamins, minerals and other nutrients present in the food, as well as other important compounds. By incorporating these cooking techniques into your meal plan, you can ensure that you get the most out of your foods and maximize the benefits to your health.

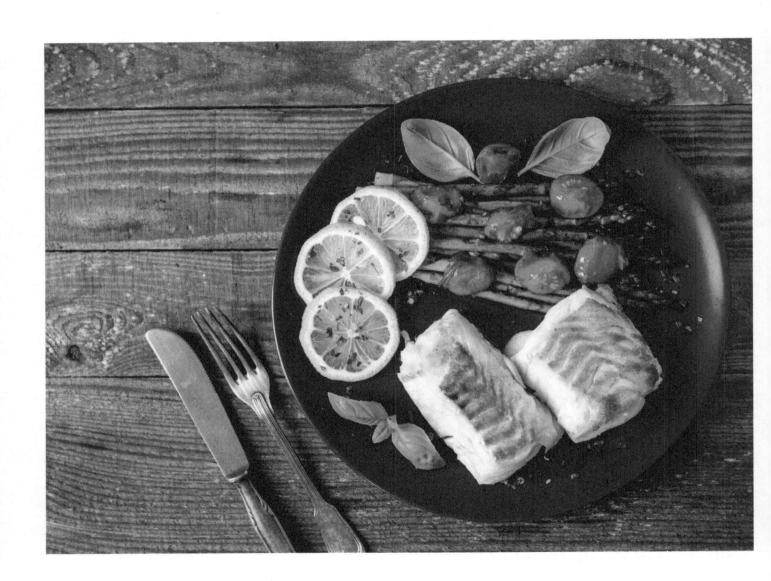

BREAKFAST RECIPES

Overnight Oats with Strawberries and Walnuts

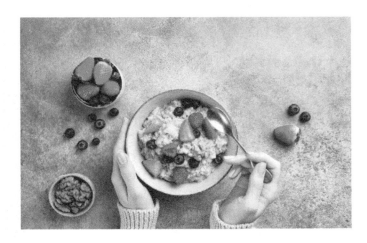

Preparation time: 10 minutes
Cooking time: None
Servings: 2

Ingredients:
- 2/3 cup rolled oats
- 2 tablespoons ground flaxseed
- 2 tablespoons chia seeds
- 2 cups unsweetened almond milk
- 1/4 teaspoon ground cinnamon
- 1/4 cup chopped walnuts
- 1/2 cup diced strawberries
- 2 tablespoons maple syrup

Directions:
1. In a medium-sized bowl, combine oats, flaxseed, chia seeds, almond milk, and cinnamon. Mix until ingredients are fully incorporated.
2. Cover the bowl and refrigerate overnight.
3. In the morning, remove the mixture from the fridge and stir in walnuts and strawberries.
4. Divide the oatmeal into two bowls and top each bowl with 1 tablespoon of maple syrup.

Nutrition values: Calories: 292; Fat: 10.5g; Carbohydrates: 39.3g; Protein: 8.5g; Fiber: 7.3g

Scrambled Egg and Vegetable Wrap

Preparation time: 10 minutes
Cooking time: 10 minutes
Servings: 2

Ingredients:
- 2 tablespoons olive oil
- 1/2 cup diced red bell pepper
- 1/2 cup diced onion
- 1/2 cup diced zucchini
- 4 large eggs
- 1/4 teaspoon sea salt
- 2 whole wheat tortillas
- 2 tablespoons chopped parsley

Directions:
1. Heat a large skillet over medium-high heat with oil.
2. Add bell pepper, onion, and zucchini, and sauté for 5 minutes.
3. In a medium-sized bowl, whisk together eggs and sea salt.
4. Pour eggs into the skillet and stir until eggs are fully cooked.
5. Heat tortillas in a dry skillet for 1 minute on each side.
6. Divide eggs among the tortillas and top with parsley.
7. Roll the tortillas and enjoy.

Nutrition values: Calories: 304; Fat: 17.7g; Carbohydrates: 21.1g; Protein: 13.3g; Fiber: 3.6g

Almond Flour Pancakes with Banana and Blueberry

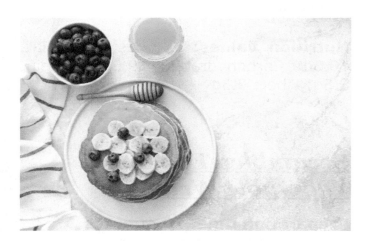

Preparation time: 10 minutes
Cooking time: 10 minutes
Servings: 2

Ingredients:
- 1/2 cup almond flour
- 1/2 teaspoon baking powder
- 1/4 teaspoon sea salt
- 1/4 teaspoon ground cinnamon
- 2 large eggs
- 1/4 cup unsweetened almond milk
- 1/2 teaspoon vanilla extract
- 1 medium banana, sliced
- 1/4 cup blueberries
- 2 tablespoons melted coconut oil

Directions:
1. In a medium-sized bowl, whisk together almond flour, baking powder, sea salt, and cinnamon.
2. In a separate bowl, whisk together eggs, almond milk, and vanilla extract.
3. Pour wet ingredients into the dry ingredients and mix until combined.
4. Heat a large non-stick skillet over medium heat. Add coconut oil.
5. Drop 1/4 cup of batter onto the skillet, then add banana slices and blueberries.
6. Cook each pancake for 2-3 minutes on each side, or until golden brown.

7. Serve pancakes with additional banana slices and blueberries.

Nutrition values: Calories: 321; Fat: 19.6g; Carbohydrates: 25.6g; Protein: 9.8g; Fiber: 5.2g

Coconut Quinoa Porridge

Preparation time: 10 minutes
Cooking time: 20 minutes
Servings: 2

Ingredients:
- 1/2 cup quinoa
- 1 cup unsweetened coconut milk
- 1/4 teaspoon ground cinnamon
- 1/4 teaspoon ground ginger
- 1/4 teaspoon ground cardamom
- 1 tablespoon maple syrup
- 1/4 cup sliced almonds
- 2 tablespoons shredded coconut
- 1/4 cup diced mango

Directions:
1. Rinse quinoa in a fine-mesh sieve.
2. In a medium-sized pot over medium heat, add quinoa, coconut milk, cinnamon, ginger, and cardamom. Bring the mixture to a simmer.
3. Reduce heat to low and cover. Simmer for 15 minutes.
4. Uncover the pot and stir in maple syrup. Simmer for an additional 5 minutes.
5. Divide the porridge into two bowls and top with almonds, coconut, and mango.

Nutrition values: Calories: 299 kcal; Fat: 12.7g; Carbohydrates: 36.4g; Protein: 7.2g; Fiber: 5.8g

Kale, Tomato, and Avocado Egg Scramble

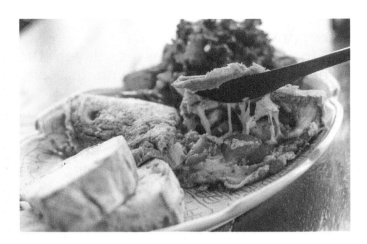

Preparation time: 10 minutes
Cooking time: 10 minutes
Servings: 4

Ingredients:
- 8 eggs
- 2 tablespoons olive oil
- 1/2 cup chopped kale
- 1/2 cup chopped tomato
- 1/2 cup chopped avocado
- 1/4 cup grated Parmesan cheese
- Salt and pepper, to taste

Directions:
1. Fry the olive oil in a big pan over medium heat.
2. Whisk the eggs together in a bowl and season with salt and pepper.
3. Pour the eggs into the skillet and cook, stirring occasionally, until the eggs are almost set.
4. Add the kale, tomato, and avocado and cook for another 1-2 minutes.
5. Sprinkle the Parmesan cheese over the top and cook for another minute.
6. Serve hot.

Nutrition values: Calories: 198, Fat: 14g, Protein: 13g, Carbs: 5g, Fiber: 2g, Sugar: 1g, Sodium: 173mg.

Sweet Potato Hash with Spinach and Feta Cheese

Preparation time: 15 minutes
Cooking time: 25 minutes
Servings: 4

Ingredients:
- 2 tablespoons olive oil
- 2 cloves garlic, minced
- 2 large sweet potatoes, peeled and diced
- ½ teaspoon ground cumin
- ½ teaspoon smoked paprika
- ¼ teaspoon ground black pepper
- 2 cups spinach, chopped
- ½ cup feta cheese, crumbled
- Salt to taste

Directions:
1. Heat oil in a large skillet over medium heat. Add garlic and cook for 30 seconds.
2. Add sweet potatoes and cook, stirring occasionally, for about 10 minutes.
3. Add cumin, smoked paprika, and black pepper, and cook for another 2 minutes.
4. Add spinach and cook for about 3 minutes, or until spinach is wilted.
5. Remove from heat and stir in feta cheese. Season with salt to taste.

Nutrition values: Calories: 159; Fat: 8g; Carbohydrates: 18g; Protein: 5g Fiber: 3.4g

Red Lentil and Zucchini Fritters

Preparation time: 10 minutes
Cooking time: 20 minutes
Servings: 8-10

Ingredients:
- 1 cup red lentils

- 2 zucchini, grated
- 1 onion, diced
- 2 cloves garlic, minced
- 1/2 cup fresh parsley, chopped
- 1 teaspoon ground cumin
- 1 teaspoon ground coriander
- 1/2 teaspoon ground cayenne pepper
- 1 teaspoon sea salt
- 1/2 cup rolled oats
- 2 tablespoons olive oil

Directions:
1.. Bring to a boil, reduce heat, and simmer for 10 minutes or until the lentils are tender. Drain and set aside.
2. Put the lentils in a pot and fill with 2 cups of water. In a large bowl, combine the grated zucchini, onion, garlic, parsley, cumin, coriander, cayenne pepper, and salt.
3. Add the cooked lentils and oats to the bowl and mix until everything is fully incorporated.
4. Heat the olive oil in a large skillet over medium heat. Using a 1/4 cup measuring cup, drop spoonfuls of the lentil mixture into the hot oil and flatten with a spatula.
5. Cook the fritters for 4-5 minutes on each side or until golden brown.
6. Serve with your favorite condiment or yogurt.

Nutrition Values (per serving): Calories: 106; Fat: 3.4g; Protein: 5.3g; Carbs: 15.3g

Yogurt Parfait with Fruit and Nuts

Preparation time: 10 minutes
Cooking time: 0 minutes
Servings: 2

Ingredients:

- 2 cups plain Greek yogurt
- 1 cup fresh berries
- 1/4 cup chopped almonds
- 1/4 cup honey

Directions:
1. In two parfait glasses, layer the Greek yogurt, berries, almonds, and honey.
2. Serve immediately or chill for later.

Nutrition Values (per serving): Calories: 531; Fat: 20g; Protein: 31g; Carbs: 57g.

Quinoa Breakfast Bowl with Berries and Almonds

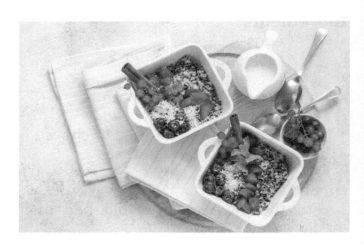

Preparation time: 10 minutes
Cooking time: 15 minutes
Servings: 2

Ingredients:
- 1 cup quinoa
- 2 cups water
- 1 cup fresh or frozen berries (raspberries, strawberries, blueberries)
- 2 tablespoons slivered almonds
- Salt and pepper, to taste
- Optional: 2 tablespoons honey or maple syrup

Directions:

1. Rinse the quinoa.
2. Bring the quinoa and water to a boil in a medium saucepan. Reduce to a simmer and cover, cooking for 15 minutes or until all the water is absorbed.
3. Once the quinoa is cooked, fluff with a fork.
4. Divide the quinoa between two bowls and top with berries and almonds.
5. Add a drizzle of honey or maple syrup, if desired.
6. Enjoy!

Nutrition values (per serving): Calories: 368; Fat: 7g; Carbohydrates: 64g; Protein: 11g Fiber: 7g; Sugar: 9g

Chia Seed Pudding with Coconut, Milk and Berries

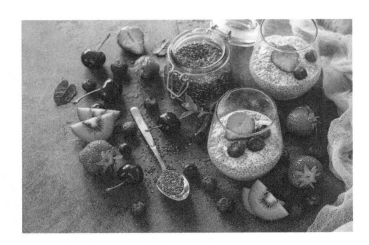

Preparation time: 10 minutes
Cooking time: None
Servings: 2

Ingredients:
- 1/2 cup chia seeds
- 2 cups coconut milk
- 1 cup fresh or frozen berries (raspberries, strawberries, blueberries, etc.)
- Optional: honey or maple syrup, to sweeten

Directions:
1. In a medium bowl, whisk together the chia seeds and coconut milk.
2. Cover the bowl and refrigerate overnight or for at least 4 hours.
3. When the chia seed pudding is set, divide it between two bowls and top with berries.
4. Add a drizzle of honey or maple syrup, if desired.
5. Enjoy!

Nutrition values: Calories: 283; Fat: 18g; Carbohydrates: 21g; Protein: 5g; Fiber: 10g; Sugar: 9g

Turmeric Latte with Coconut Milk

Preparation time: 5 minutes
Cooking time: 5 minutes
Servings: 1

Ingredients:
- 1 cup coconut milk
- 1 teaspoon ground turmeric
- 1 teaspoon ground ginger
- 1/2 teaspoon ground cinnamon
- 1 teaspoon honey (or maple syrup)

Directions:
1. In a small saucepan, heat the coconut milk over medium heat until it is steaming.
2. Add the turmeric, ginger, cinnamon and honey. Mix until all the ingredients are blended.
3. Continue to heat the mixture for another 2-3 minutes or until it is hot and fragrant.
4. Pour the latte into a mug. Enjoy.

Nutrition Values: Calories: 142; Fat: 11.5g; Carbohydrates: 11.5g; Protein: 2.5g; Fiber: 2g; Sugar: 8.5g

Avocado toast with poached egg

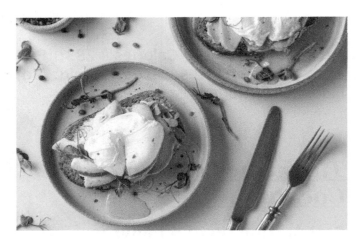

Preparation time: 5 minutes
Cooking time: 10 minutes
Servings: 2

Ingredients:
*   2 slices of whole grain bread
*   1 ripe avocado
*   1 tablespoon of olive oil
*   2 poached eggs
*   Salt and pepper to taste

Directions:
1. Toast the bread slices in a toaster or in a preheated oven at 350 degrees for 5 minutes.
2. Meanwhile, cut the avocado in half and scoop out the flesh into a bowl. Mash it with a fork and season it with salt, pepper and olive oil.
3. Spread the avocado mash over the bread slices.
4. Poach the eggs in a pot of simmering water for 5 minutes.
5. Place the poached eggs on top of the avocado toast.

6. Serve immediately.

Nutrition values: Calories: 389; Total Fat: 20g; Saturated Fat: 3g; Cholesterol: 186 mg; Sodium: 229 mg; Protein: 11 g

Acai Bowl with Hemp Seeds

Preparation Time: 10 minutes
Cooking Time: 0 minutes
Servings: 1

Ingredients:
*   ½ cup frozen acai berries
*   ½ banana
*   ¼ cup unsweetened almond milk
*   1 teaspoon honey
*   1 tablespoon hemp seeds
*   1 teaspoon chia seeds
*   Toppings of your choice (granola, fresh fruit, coconut flakes, etc.)

Directions:
1. Add the acai berries, banana, almond milk, honey, and hemp seeds to a blender and blend until smooth.
2. Pour the smoothie into a bowl and add the chia seeds.
3. Top with your desired toppings and enjoy!

Nutrition Values: Calories: 315; Fat: 10g; Carbohydrates: 46g; Protein: 8g

Smoked Salmon and Spinach Frittata

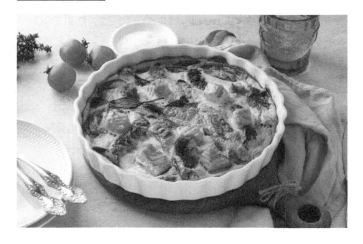

Preparation Time: 10 minutes
Cooking Time: 20 minutes
Servings: 4

Ingredients:
*   2 tablespoons olive oil
*   1 ½ cups chopped onion
*   4 cups baby spinach
*   ¼ teaspoon salt
*   8 large eggs
*   4 ounces smoked salmon, chopped
*   ½ cup feta cheese, crumbled

Directions:
1. Preheat oven to 350°F.
2. Heat the olive oil in a large oven-safe skillet over medium heat.
3. Add the onion and sauté for 5 minutes.
4. Add the spinach and salt and cook for another 2 minutes.
5. In a medium bowl, whisk together the eggs and salmon.
6. Pour the egg mixture over the spinach and onion in the skillet.
7. Sprinkle the feta cheese over the top.
8. Bake for 15-20 minutes, or until the eggs are set.
9. Slice and serve.

Nutrition Values: Calories: 188; Fat: 12g; Carbohydrates: 4g; Protein: 16g

Breakfast Burrito with Sweet Potato and Black Beans

Preparation Time: 10 minutes
Cooking Time: 15 minutes
Servings: 4

Ingredients:
*   2 tablespoons olive oil
*   1 cup diced sweet potato
*   1 cup black beans, rinsed and drained
*   4 large eggs
*   ¼ teaspoon garlic powder
*   Salt and pepper, to taste
*   4 whole-wheat tortillas
*   ¼ cup shredded cheddar cheese
*   Salsa, for serving

Directions:
1. Heat a large skillet over medium-high heat with oil.
2. Insert the sweet potato and simmer for 5 minutes, stirring occasionally.
3. Add the black beans and cook for another 5 minutes.
4. In a medium bowl, whisk together the eggs, garlic powder, salt, and pepper.
5. Pour the egg mixture into the skillet and scramble until the eggs are cooked.
6. Divide the egg mixture among the tortillas.
7. Top with the cheese and salsa.
8. Roll up and serve.

Nutrition Values: Calories: 317; Fat: 15g; Carbohydrates: 25g; Protein: 17g

Banana Oat Smoothie Bowl

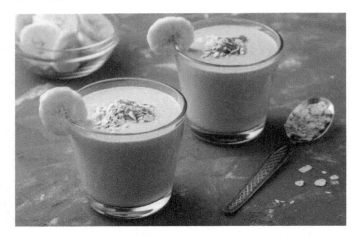

Preparation Time: 10 minutes
Cooking Time: 0 minutes
Servings: 1

Ingredients:
- 1 banana
- ½ cup rolled oats
- ¼ cup unsweetened almond milk
- 1 tablespoon honey
- Toppings of your choice (granola, fresh fruit, coconut flakes, etc.)

Directions:
1. Add the banana, oats, almond milk, and honey to a blender and blend until smooth.
2. Pour the smoothie into a bowl and add your desired toppings.
3. Enjoy!

Nutrition Values: Calories: 397; Fat: 5g; Carbohydrates: 74g; Protein: 9g

Poached Egg with Asparagus and Tomatoes

Preparation Time: 10 minutes
Cooking Time: 8 minutes
Servings: 2

Ingredients:
- 2 large eggs
- 1/2 cup asparagus, chopped
- 1/2 cup cherry tomatoes, halved
- 2 tsp olive oil
- Salt and pepper, to taste
- 2 tsp fresh parsley, chopped

Directions:
1. Fill a medium saucepan with 1 inch of water and bring to a gentle simmer.
2. Add the chopped asparagus and tomatoes to the simmering water and cook for 3 minutes.
3. Gently lower the eggs into the saucepan and cook for 5 minutes.
4. Remove the eggs and vegetables from the heat and transfer to a plate.
5. Drizzle with olive oil and sprinkle with salt, pepper, and parsley.

Nutrition Values: Calories: 188; Fat: 11.5g; Carbohydrates: 5.5g; Protein: 12.5g; Sodium: 367mg; Fiber: 2.5g

Buckwheat Porridge with Apple and Cinnamon

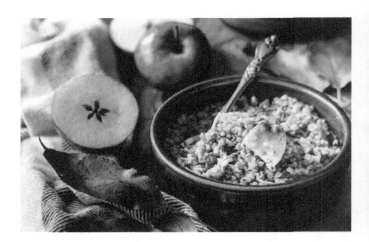

Preparation Time: 5 minutes
Cooking Time: 15 minutes
Servings: 2

Ingredients:

- 1 cup buckwheat groats
- 2 cups water
- 1/2 cup diced apple
- 1/2 tsp ground cinnamon
- 1 tsp honey

Directions:
1. Place the buckwheat groats and water in a medium saucepan and bring to a boil.
2. Reduce the heat and simmer for 10 minutes, stirring occasionally.
3. Add the diced apple, cinnamon, and honey and cook for an additional 5 minutes.
4. Serve warm and enjoy.

Nutrition Values: Calories: 320; Fat: 4g; Carbohydrates: 63g; Protein: 12g; Sodium: 9mg; Fiber: 10 g

Omelet with Spinach, Mushrooms, and Feta

Preparation Time: 15 minutes
Cooking Time: 10 minutes
Servings: 2

Ingredients:
- 2 tsp olive oil
- 1/2 cup mushrooms, sliced
- 1/2 cup spinach, chopped
- 2 large eggs
- 2 tbsp feta cheese, crumbled
- Salt and pepper, to taste

Directions:
1. Heat the olive oil in a large non-stick skillet.
2. Add the mushrooms and spinach and cook for 5 minutes, stirring often.
3. In a bowl, whisk together the eggs and season with salt and pepper.
4. Reduce the heat to low and pour the egg mixture into the pan.
5. Cook for 3 minutes, stirring frequently.

6. Sprinkle the feta cheese over the omelet and continue to cook for 2 minutes.
7. Serve immediately and enjoy.

Nutrition Values: Calories: 191; Fat: 12.7g; Carbohydrates: 4.3g; Protein: 14.3g; Sodium: 293mg; Fiber: 1.7g

Gluten-Free Fruit and Nut Granola

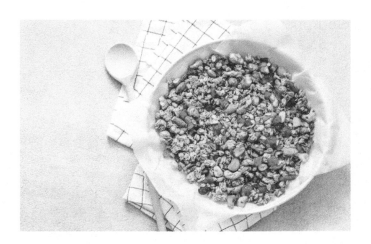

Preparation Time: 5 minutes
Cooking Time: 30 minutes
Servings 8

Ingredients:
- 2 cups gluten-free rolled oats
- 1/2 cup almonds, chopped
- 1/2 cup walnuts, chopped
- 1/2 cup dried cranberries
- 2 tbsp chia seeds
- 1/4 cup coconut oil, melted
- 2 tbsp honey
- 1/2 tsp ground cinnamon

Directions:
1. Preheat the oven to 350°F.
2. In a large bowl, mix together the oats, almonds, walnuts, cranberries, and chia seeds.

3. In a small bowl, mix together the melted coconut oil, honey, and cinnamon.

4. Pour the wet ingredients into the dry ingredients and mix until everything is evenly coated.

5. Spread the granola onto a parchment paper-lined baking sheet and bake for 30 minutes, stirring occasionally.

6. Allow the granola to cool before serving.

Nutrition Values:
Calories: 244; Fat: 16.1 g; Carbohydrates: 24.7 g; Protein: 6 g; Sodium: 3.5 mg; Fiber: 5.2 g

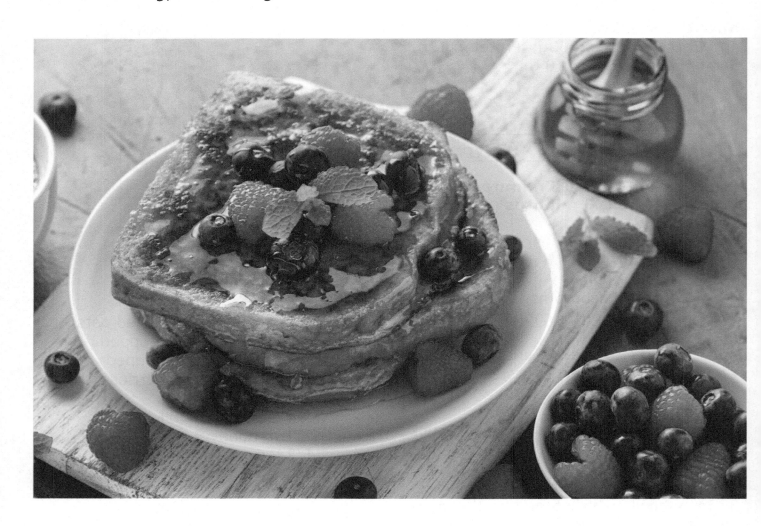

POULTRY AND MEAT RECIPES

Slow Cooker Pulled Chicken with Sweet Potatoes

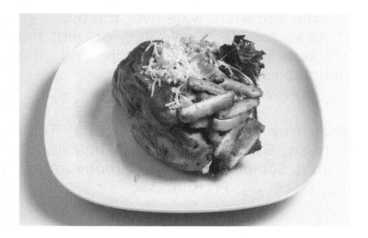

Preparation time: 10 minutes
Cooking time: 4 hours
Servings: 4

Ingredients:
* 4 boneless, skinless chicken breasts
* 1 large sweet potato, peeled and diced
* 1/2 cup chicken broth
* 1 tbsp olive oil
* 1/2 tsp garlic powder
* 1/2 tsp onion powder
* 1/4 tsp paprika
* Salt and pepper to taste

Directions:
1. Place chicken breasts in the bottom of a slow cooker.
2. Top with diced sweet potato.
3. In a small bowl, combine chicken broth, olive oil, garlic powder, onion powder, and paprika. Pour over chicken and sweet potato.

4. Cover and cook on low for 4 hours or until chicken is cooked through and sweet potato is tender.
5. Remove chicken from slow cooker and shred it.
6. Return shredded chicken to slow cooker and stir to combine.
7. Serve with your favorite side dishes.

Nutrition values: Calories: 296, Fat: 10g; Carbohydrates: 15g; Protein: 30g

Grilled Beef and Broccoli Stir-Fry

Preparation time: 10 minutes
Cooking time: 10 minutes
Servings: 4

Ingredients:
* 1 pound sirloin steak, cut into thin strips
* 1 tablespoon olive oil
* 1 onion, diced
* 2 cloves garlic, minced
* 2 cups broccoli florets
* 2 tablespoons soy sauce
* 2 tablespoons honey
* 1 teaspoon ground ginger
* 1 teaspoon red pepper flakes

Directions:
1. Heat a large skillet or wok over medium-high heat.
2. Add the steak strips and olive oil and cook for 3-4 minutes, stirring frequently, until the steak is cooked through.
3. Add the onion and garlic and cook for another 2 minutes.
4. Add the broccoli and cook for 3 minutes, stirring frequently.
5. In a small bowl, mix together the soy sauce, honey, ginger and red pepper flakes. Pour the mixture over the steak and vegetables and stir to combine.

6. Cook for an additional 2 minutes, stirring frequently, until the sauce has thickened and the vegetables are tender.
7. Serve warm.

Nutrition values: Calories: 310; Total Fat: 10g; Saturated Fat: 2g; Cholesterol: 65mg; Sodium: 789mg; Carbohydrates: 21g; Fiber: 3g; Protein: 33g

Baked Chicken Breasts with Mushrooms and Herbs

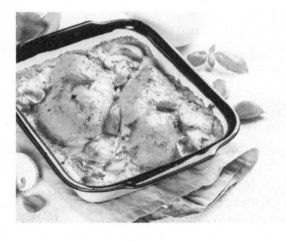

Preparation time: 10 minutes
Cooking time: 25 minutes
Servings: 4

Ingredients:
• 4 boneless, skinless chicken breasts
• 1 tablespoon olive oil
• 1 onion, diced
• 8 ounces mushrooms, sliced
• 2 cloves garlic, minced
• 1 teaspoon dried oregano
• 1 teaspoon dried thyme
• 1 teaspoon dried basil
• 1 teaspoon salt
• 1 teaspoon black pepper
• 1/4 cup white wine

Directions:
1. Preheat oven to 350°F.
2. Heat a large skillet over medium-high heat. Add the olive oil, onion, mushrooms and garlic and cook for 5 minutes, stirring frequently, until the vegetables are softened.
3. Put the chicken breasts in a saucepan. Top with the cooked vegetables and sprinkle with oregano, thyme, basil, salt and pepper.
4. Pour the white wine over the top.
5. Bake for 20-25 minutes, or until the chicken is cooked through and the vegetables are tender.
6. Serve warm.

Nutrition values: Calories: 270; Total Fat: 8g; Saturated Fat: 1g; Cholesterol: 73mg; Sodium: 554mg; Carbohydrates: 7g; Fiber: 2g; Protein: 33g

Grilled Sirloin Steak with Avocado Salsa

Preparation time: 10 minutes
Cooking time: 10 minutes
Servings: 4

Ingredients:
• 2 pounds sirloin steak
• 1 tablespoon olive oil
• 1 teaspoon garlic powder
• 1 teaspoon onion powder
• 1 teaspoon dried oregano
• 1 teaspoon salt
• 1 teaspoon black pepper
• 1 avocado, diced
• 1/4 cup chopped cilantro
• 1/4 cup diced red onion
• 1 jalapeno, seeded and diced
• 2 tablespoons lime juice

Directions:
1. Heat a grill over high heat.

2. Rub the steak with olive oil and sprinkle with garlic powder, onion powder, oregano, salt and pepper.
3. Cook the steak for 5-6 minutes per side, or until cooked to desired doneness.
4. In a small bowl, mix together the avocado, cilantro, red onion, jalapeno and lime juice.
5. Serve the steak with the avocado salsa.

Nutrition values: Calories: 375; Total Fat: 18g; Saturated Fat: 5g; Cholesterol: 107mg; Sodium: 567mg; Carbohydrates: 5g; Fiber: 3g; Protein: 41g

Slow Cooker Chicken and Rice Soup

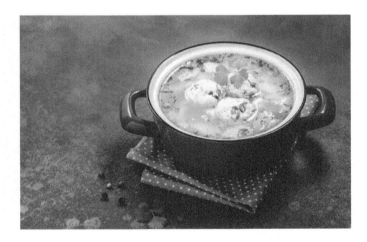

Preparation time: 10 minutes
Cooking time: 4-6 hours
Servings: 8

Ingredients:
- 2 tablespoons olive oil
- 2 cloves garlic, minced
- 1 onion, diced
- 2 cups diced carrots
- 2 cups diced celery
- 1 teaspoon Italian seasoning
- Salt and pepper, to taste

- 4 cups chicken broth
- 4 cups water
- 2 cups cooked, diced chicken
- 1 cup uncooked long grain white rice

Directions:
1. Heat the olive oil in a skillet over medium heat.
2. Add the garlic, onion, carrots, celery, Italian seasoning, salt, and pepper and cook until the vegetables are tender, about 5 minutes.
3. Transfer the vegetables to a slow cooker.
4. Add the chicken broth, water, chicken, and rice to the slow cooker and stir to combine.
5. Cook on low heat for 4-6 hours, until the rice is cooked through.

Nutrition values: Calories: 230 kcal; Fat: 6 g; Carbohydrates: 21 g; Protein: 18g

Grilled Chicken Burgers with Pesto

Preparation time: 10 minutes
Cooking time: 20 minutes
Servings: 4

Ingredients:
- 2 lb. ground chicken
- 1/2 cup Pesto
- 2 cloves garlic, minced
- 1/2 teaspoon salt
- 1/4 teaspoon black pepper
- 4 whole wheat hamburger buns

Directions:
1. Preheat grill to medium-high heat.
2. In a large bowl, combine the chicken, pesto, garlic, salt and pepper. Mix until just combined.
3. Form the mixture into 4 equal patties.

4. Place the patties on the preheated grill and cook for 8-10 minutes per side, or until the chicken is cooked through.
5. Serve the burgers on the whole wheat buns and enjoy!

Nutrition values (Per Serving):
Calories: 350; Fat: 16g; Carbohydrates: 17g; Protein: 31g

Grilled Flank Steak with Chimichurri Sauce

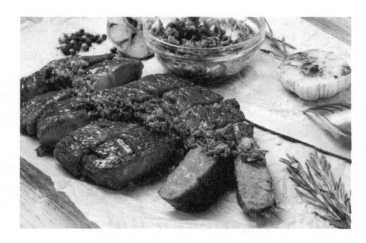

Preparation time: 10 minutes
Cooking time: 10 minutes
Servings: 4

Ingredients:
*   1 pound flank steak
*   2 tablespoons olive oil
*   1 teaspoon sea salt
*   1 teaspoon freshly ground pepper
*   1/2 cup freshly chopped parsley
*   1/4 cup freshly chopped oregano
*   2 cloves garlic, minced
*   2 tablespoons red wine vinegar
*   1/4 cup extra-virgin olive oil

Directions:
1. Heat a grill pan over medium-high heat.
2. Rub olive oil over flank steak and season with salt and pepper.

3. Grill the steak for about 5 minutes per side or until desired doneness is achieved.
4. Meanwhile, in a medium bowl, mix together the parsley, oregano, garlic, red wine vinegar, and extra-virgin olive oil to make the chimichurri sauce.
5. Let the steak rest for 5 minutes, then slice into thin strips.
6. Serve the steak with the chimichurri sauce.

Nutrition Values (per serving):
Calories: 393; Fat: 30.9g; Carbohydrates: 1.2g; Protein: 28.3g;

Slow Cooker Chicken and Veggie Stew

Preparation time: 10 minutes
Cooking time: 6-7 hours
Servings: 8

Ingredients:
*   2 tablespoons olive oil
*   2 boneless, skinless chicken breasts
*   1 onion, chopped
*   2 cloves garlic, minced
*   2 carrots, chopped
*   2 celery stalks, chopped
*   2 cups low-sodium chicken broth
*   1 teaspoon dried oregano
*   1 teaspoon dried basil
*   ½ teaspoon dried rosemary
*   ¼ teaspoon salt
*   ¼ teaspoon black pepper
*   1 (14.5-ounce) can diced tomatoes
*   1 (15-ounce) can cannellini beans, rinsed and drained
*   1 cup frozen peas
*   2 tablespoons chopped fresh parsley

Directions:

1. Heat oil in a large skillet over medium-high heat. Add chicken and cook until golden brown, about 2 minutes per side. Remove chicken from skillet and transfer to a slow cooker.

2. Add onion, garlic, carrots, and celery to the skillet and cook, stirring occasionally, until vegetables are slightly softened, about 5 minutes. Transfer vegetables to the slow cooker.

3. Pour chicken broth over the chicken and vegetables in the slow cooker. Add oregano, basil, rosemary, salt, and pepper. Stir to combine.

4. Cover slow cooker and cook on low heat for 6-7 hours.

5. Add tomatoes, cannellini beans, and peas to the slow cooker and stir to combine. Cover and cook on high heat for an additional 15 minutes.

6. Serve stew topped with fresh parsley.

Nutrition Values: Calories: 205; Fat: 6g; Carbohydrates: 18g; Protein: 19g; Fiber: 5g

Grilled Pork Tenderloin with Roasted Vegetables

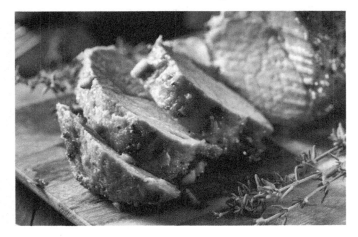

Preparation time: 10 minutes
Cooking time: 30 minutes
Servings: 4

Ingredients:
- 2 tablespoons olive oil

- 2 pork tenderloins (1 pound each)
- Salt and black pepper to taste
- 2 red bell peppers, sliced
- 1 onion, chopped
- 2 cloves garlic, minced
- 1 teaspoon dried oregano
- 1 teaspoon dried basil
- 1 teaspoon dried rosemary
- ½ teaspoon red pepper flakes

Directions:
1. Preheat grill to medium-high heat.
2. Brush pork tenderloins with 1 tablespoon of olive oil and season with salt and pepper.
3. Place pork on the grill and cook for 5 minutes per side.
4. In a large bowl, combine red bell peppers, onion, garlic, oregano, basil, rosemary, red pepper flakes, and remaining tablespoon of olive oil. Toss to combine.
5. Place vegetables on the grill and cook for 15 minutes, stirring occasionally.
6. Remove pork and vegetables from the grill and let rest for 5 minutes before slicing pork and serving with vegetables.

Nutrition Values: Calories: 321; Fat: 13g; Carbohydrates: 10g; Protein: 37g; Fiber: 3g

Grilled Lamb Chops with Mango Salsa

Preparation time: 10 minutes
Cooking time: 10 minutes
Servings: 4

Ingredients:
- 4 lamb chops
- Salt and black pepper to taste
- 2 tablespoons olive oil
- ½ mango, diced
- ½ red onion, diced
- 1 jalapeno pepper, seeded and diced

23

- 2 tablespoons chopped fresh cilantro
- 2 tablespoons fresh lime juice

Directions:
1. Preheat grill to medium-high heat.
2. Brush lamb chops with 1 tablespoon of olive oil and season with salt and pepper.
3. Place lamb chops on the grill and cook for 5 minutes per side.
4. In a medium bowl, combine mango, red onion, jalapeno pepper, cilantro, and lime juice. Toss to combine.
5. Drizzle remaining tablespoon of olive oil over mango salsa and stir to combine.
6. Serve grilled lamb chops with mango salsa.

Nutrition Values:
Calories: 209; Fat: 13g; Carbohydrates: 8g; Protein: 14g; Fiber: 1g

Slow Cooker Beef and Barley Stew

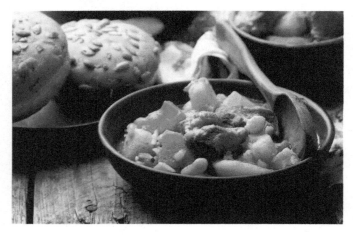

Preparation time: 10 minutes
Cooking time: 8-10 hours
Servings: 6

Ingredients:
- 2 tablespoons olive oil
- 1 pound stew beef, cut into 1-inch cubes

- Salt and black pepper to taste
- 1 onion, chopped
- 2 cloves garlic, minced
- 2 carrots, chopped
- 2 celery stalks, chopped
- 2 cups low-sodium beef broth
- 1 teaspoon dried oregano
- 1 teaspoon dried basil
- ½ teaspoon dried rosemary
- ¼ teaspoon salt
- ¼ teaspoon black pepper
- 1 (15 ounce) can diced tomatoes
- 1 cup pearl barley
- 2 tablespoons chopped fresh parsley

Directions:
1. Heat oil in a large skillet over medium-high heat. Add beef and cook until browned, about 2 minutes per side.
2. Transfer beef to a slow cooker. Add onion, garlic, carrots, and celery to the skillet and cook, stirring occasionally, until vegetables are slightly softened, about 5 minutes. Transfer vegetables to the slow cooker.
3. Pour beef broth over the beef and vegetables in the slow cooker. Add oregano, basil, rosemary, salt, and pepper. Stir to combine.
4. Cover slow cooker and cook on low heat for 8-10 hours.
5. Add tomatoes, barley, and parsley to the slow cooker and stir to combine. Cover and cook on high heat for an additional 15 minutes.
6. Serve stew topped with fresh parsley.

Nutrition Values: Calories: 291; Fat: 8g; Carbohydrates: 25g; Protein: 28g; Fiber: 4g

Baked Chicken Thighs with Apples and Onions

Preparation Time: 10 minutes
Cooking Time: 40 minutes

Servings: 4
Ingredients:
- 4 boneless, skinless chicken thighs
- 2 apples, diced
- 1 onion, diced
- 1 tablespoon extra-virgin olive oil
- 1 tablespoon dried oregano
- 1/2 teaspoon garlic powder
- 1/2 teaspoon sea salt
- 1/4 teaspoon black pepper

Directions:
1. Preheat oven to 375°F.
2. In a medium bowl, combine chicken thighs, apples, onion, olive oil, oregano, garlic powder, salt and pepper.
3. Transfer mixture to a 9x13-inch baking dish and spread out evenly.
4. Bake for 40 minutes, or until chicken is cooked through and apples and onions are tender.

Nutrition Values: Calories: 212; Fat: 9g; Carbohydrates: 12g; Protein: 21g Sodium: 283mg

Grilled Turkey Breast with Honey Mustard

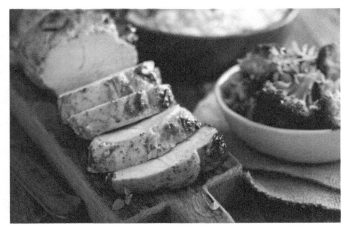

Preparation Time: 20 minutes
Cooking Time: 20 minutes
Servings: 4

Ingredients:

- 4 boneless, skinless turkey breasts
- 1/4 cup Dijon mustard
- 3 tablespoons honey
- 1 tablespoon extra-virgin olive oil
- 1 teaspoon garlic powder
- 1/2 teaspoon sea salt
- 1/4 teaspoon black pepper

Directions:
1. Preheat grill to medium-high heat.
2. In a small bowl, stir together mustard, honey, olive oil, garlic powder, salt and pepper.
3. Brush mixture over the turkey breasts.
4. Put the turkey on the grill and cook it for 12 minutes. Flip, brush with more of the mustard mixture and cook for 10 minutes, or until cooked through.

Nutrition Values: Calories: 210; Fat: 5g; Carbohydrates: 10g; Protein: 28g; Sodium: 461mg

Slow Cooker Chicken Cacciatore

Preparation Time: 15 minutes
Cooking Time: 6 hours
Servings: 6

Ingredients:
- 4 boneless, skinless chicken breasts
- 1 onion, diced
- 2 cloves garlic, minced
- 1 red bell pepper, diced
- 1 green bell pepper, diced
- 1 can (14.5 ounces) diced tomatoes
- 1 can (8 ounces) tomato sauce
- 1 tablespoon Italian seasoning
- 1 teaspoon sea salt
- 1/2 teaspoon black pepper

Directions:

1. Place chicken, onion, garlic, bell peppers, diced tomatoes, tomato sauce, Italian seasoning, salt and pepper in a slow cooker and stir to combine.
2. Cover and cook on low heat for 6 hours.

Nutrition Values: Calories: 226; Fat: 5g; Carbohydrates: 20g; Protein: 25g; Sodium: 1075mg

Grilled Bison Burgers with Avocado

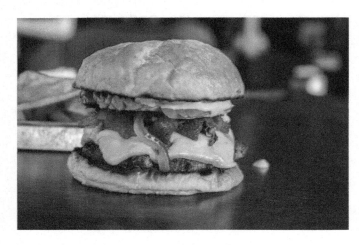

Preparation Time: 10 minutes
Cooking Time: 10 minutes
Servings: 4

Ingredients:
- 1 pound ground bison
- 1/4 cup diced onion
- 1/4 teaspoon sea salt
- 1/4 teaspoon black pepper
- 1/4 teaspoon garlic powder
- 1/4 teaspoon smoked paprika
- 1 avocado, sliced
- 4 whole-grain hamburger buns

Directions:
1. Preheat grill to medium-high heat.

2. In a medium bowl, combine bison, onion, salt, pepper, garlic powder and smoked paprika. Form the mixture into 4 patties.
3. Grill the burgers for 5 minutes per side, or until cooked through.
4. Serve the burgers on the buns topped with the avocado slices.

Nutrition Values: Calories: 339; Fat: 18g; Carbohydrates: 22g; Protein: 24g; Sodium: 299mg

Grilled Pork Chops with Pineapple Salsa

Preparation time: 10 minutes
Cooking time: 10 minutes
Servings: 4

Ingredients:
- 4 (1-inch-thick) pork chops
- 1 cup diced fresh pineapple
- 1/4 cup diced red onion
- 1 jalapeno pepper, seeded and minced
- 2 tablespoons chopped fresh cilantro
- 2 tablespoons lime juice
- 1 teaspoon olive oil
- 1/2 teaspoon ground cumin
- Salt and freshly ground black pepper

Directions:
1. Preheat an outdoor grill or indoor grill pan to medium-high heat.
2. Brush pork chops with olive oil and season with salt, pepper and cumin.
3. Grill pork chops for 5 minutes per side or until cooked through.
4. Meanwhile, in a medium bowl, mix together pineapple, onion, jalapeno pepper, cilantro, lime juice, and olive oil.
5. Serve pork chops topped with pineapple salsa.

Nutrition values: Calories: 263; Total Fat: 8.8g; Saturated Fat: 2.7g; Cholesterol: 80mg; Sodium: 66mg; Carbohydrates: 11.4g; Fiber: 1g; Sugar: 8.4g; Protein: 27.2g

Slow Cooker Beef and Bean Chili

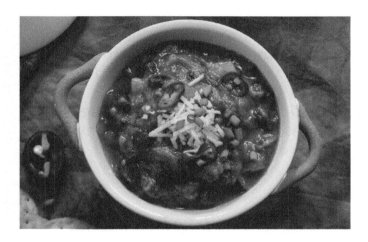

Preparation time: 10 minutes
Cooking time: 4 hours
Servings: 6

Ingredients:
• 1 lb. lean ground beef
• 1 onion, diced
• 2 cloves garlic, minced
• 1 can (14.5 oz) diced tomatoes
• 1 can (15 oz) black beans, drained and rinsed
• 1 can (15 oz) kidney beans, drained and rinsed
• 1 cup vegetable broth
• 2 tablespoons chili powder
• 1 teaspoon ground cumin
• 1 teaspoon oregano
• 1/2 teaspoon salt
• 1/4 teaspoon black pepper

Directions:

1. In a large skillet, cook ground beef over medium heat until browned. Drain fat and transfer to a crockpot.
2. Add onion, garlic, tomatoes, black beans, kidney beans, vegetable broth, chili powder, cumin, oregano, salt, and pepper to the slow cooker. Stir to combine.
3. Cover and cook on low heat for 4 hours.
4. Serve chili with desired toppings.

Nutrition values:
Calories: 358; Total Fat: 7.2g; Saturated Fat: 2.6g; Cholesterol: 55mg; Sodium: 798mg; Carbohydrates: 47.5g; Fiber: 13.5g; Sugar: 7.2g; Protein: 27.5g

Baked Lemon-Garlic Chicken

Preparation time: 15 minutes
Cooking time: 25 minutes
Servings: 4

Ingredients:
• 4 boneless skinless chicken breasts
• 2 tablespoons olive oil
• 3 cloves garlic, minced
• 2 tablespoons fresh lemon juice
• 1 teaspoon dried oregano
• 1 teaspoon dried basil
• Salt and pepper to taste

Directions:
1. Preheat oven to 400°F. Lightly grease a baking dish.
2. In a small bowl, whisk together olive oil, garlic, lemon juice, oregano, basil, salt, and pepper.
3. Place chicken in the baking dish and coat with the lemon-garlic mixture. Bake for 25 minutes or until chicken is cooked through and lightly browned.

Nutrition values: Calories: 297 kcal; Fat: 10.8g; Carbohydrates: 2.7g; Protein: 44.7g

Coconut Curry Chicken

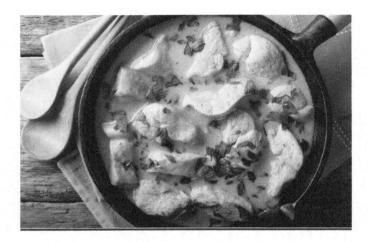

Preparation time: 10 minutes
Cooking time: 25 minutes
Servings: 4

Ingredients:
• 4 boneless chicken breasts
• 2 cloves of garlic, chopped
• 1 tablespoon of fresh ginger, minced
• 1 tablespoon of coconut oil
• 1 teaspoon of ground cumin
• 1 teaspoon of ground coriander
• 1 teaspoon of turmeric
• 1 teaspoon of ground black pepper
• 1 teaspoon of sea salt
• 1 can of coconut milk
• 1 cup of white basmati rice
• 1 cup of frozen green peas
• 1 tablespoon of fresh cilantro, chopped

Directions:
1. Preheat the oven to 350 degrees.

2. In a large bowl, combine the chicken breasts, garlic, ginger, coconut oil, cumin, coriander, turmeric, black pepper and sea salt. Mix the ingredients together until well combined.
3. Place the chicken in an oven-safe dish and bake for 20-25 minutes.
4. In a large pot, bring the coconut milk to a boil. Add the rice and frozen green peas, reduce the heat, and simmer for 10-15 minutes.
5. Once the chicken is cooked through, remove from the oven and slice into strips.
6. Divide the cooked rice and peas between four plates. Top with the sliced chicken and garnish with cilantro.

Nutrition Values (per serving): Calories: 324; Fat: 9g; Carbohydrates: 30g; Protein: 30g

Grilled Teriyaki Chicken

Preparation time: 10 minutes
Cooking time: 15 minutes
Servings: 4

Ingredients:
• ½ cup low-sodium soy sauce
• ¼ cup honey
• 2 cloves garlic, minced
• 1 teaspoon freshly grated ginger
• 1 teaspoon sesame oil
• ½ teaspoon red pepper flakes
• 4 boneless skinless chicken breasts

Directions:
1. In a small bowl, whisk together soy sauce, honey, garlic, ginger, sesame oil, and red pepper flakes.
2. Place chicken in a shallow dish and coat with the teriyaki sauce. Cover and let marinate for at least 10 minutes.

3. Heat grill to medium-high heat. Grill chicken for about 8 minutes per side or until cooked through.

Nutrition values: Calories: 266 kcal; Fat: 5.3g; Carbohydrates: 17.6g; Protein: 37.4g

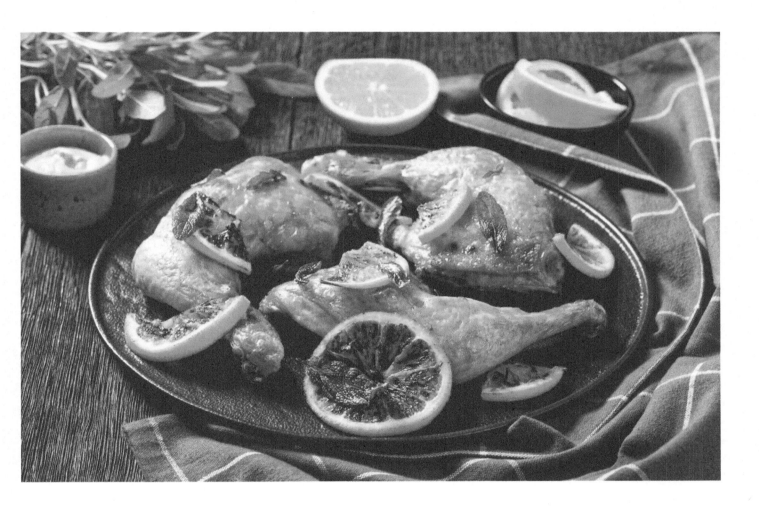

FISH AND SEAFOOD RECIPES

Grilled Salmon with Dill and Garlic

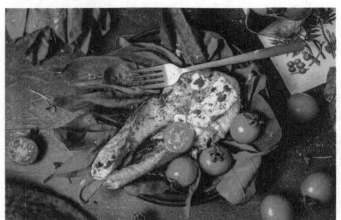

Preparation time: 15 minutes
Cooking time: 8 minutes
Servings: 4
Ingredients:
* 4 Salmon fillets, 4-6 ounces each
* 2 tablespoons olive oil
* 2 cloves garlic, minced
* 1 tablespoon fresh dill, chopped
* 1 teaspoon kosher salt
* 1/4 teaspoon black pepper

Directions:
1. Preheat an outdoor grill or grill pan over medium heat.
2. In a small bowl, mix together the olive oil, garlic, dill, salt, and pepper.
3. Rub the mixture onto the salmon fillets.
4. Place the salmon on the grill and cook for 4-5 minutes per side, or until cooked through.
5. Serve the grilled salmon with additional dill and freshly cracked black pepper.

Nutrition values: Calories: 287; Fat: 17g; Carbohydrates: 0g; Protein: 35g

Salmon and Asparagus in Foil Packets

Preparation time: 10 minutes
Cooking time: 20 minutes
Servings: 4
Ingredients:
* 4 salmon fillets, 4-6 ounces each
* 1 pound asparagus, trimmed
* 4 cloves garlic, minced
* 2 tablespoons olive oil
* 1 teaspoon kosher salt
* 1/4 teaspoon black pepper

Directions:
1. Preheat oven to 400°F and cut four pieces of aluminum foil, each about 12-inches long.
2. Divide the salmon, asparagus, and garlic between the four pieces of foil.
3. Drizzle the olive oil over the salmon and asparagus and season with salt and pepper.
4. Fold the aluminum foil into packets and place on a baking sheet.
5. Bake in the preheated oven for 20 minutes or until the salmon is cooked through.

Nutrition values: Calories: 306; Fat: 16g; Carbohydrates: 8g; Protein: 33g

Baked Salmon with Lemon and Herbs

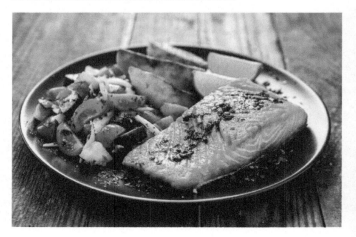

Preparation time: 10 minutes
Cooking time: 15 minutes
Servings: 4

Ingredients:
- 4 salmon fillets, 4-6 ounces each
- 2 tablespoons olive oil
- 2 cloves garlic, minced
- 2 tablespoons fresh lemon juice
- 2 tablespoons fresh herbs (such as thyme, rosemary, or oregano), chopped
- 1 teaspoon kosher salt
- 1/4 teaspoon black pepper

Directions:
1. Preheat oven to 400°F.
2. Place the salmon fillets in a baking dish.
3. In a small bowl, mix together the olive oil, garlic, lemon juice, herbs, salt, and pepper.
4. Pour the mixture over the salmon and use a spoon to spread it evenly.
5. Bake in preheated oven for 15 minutes or until the salmon is cooked through.

Nutrition values: Calories: 294; Fat: 18g; Carbohydrates: 1g; Protein: 35g

Pan-Fried Salmon with Spinach and Tomatoes

Preparation time: 10 minutes
Cooking time: 8 minutes
Servings: 4

Ingredients:
- 4 salmon fillets, 4-6 ounces each
- 2 tablespoons olive oil
- 2 cloves garlic, minced
- 2 cups baby spinach
- 1 cup cherry tomatoes, halved
- 1/2 teaspoon kosher salt
- 1/4 teaspoon black pepper

Directions:
1. Fry the olive oil in a big pan over medium heat.
2. Add the garlic, baby spinach, and cherry tomatoes.
3. Cook, stirring frequently, for 2-3 minutes.
4. Add the salmon fillets to the skillet and season with salt and pepper.
5. Cook for 4-5 minutes per side, or until the salmon is cooked through.
6. Serve the salmon over the spinach and tomatoes.

Nutrition values: Calories: 305; Fat: 17g; Carbohydrates: 5g; Protein: 33g

Baked Halibut with Garlic and Parsley

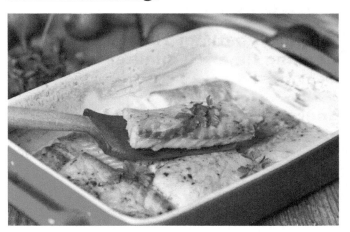

Preparation time: 10 minutes
Cooking time: 20 minutes
Servings: 4

Ingredients:
- 4 (6-ounce) halibut fillets
- 1/4 teaspoon freshly ground black pepper
- 1/4 teaspoon salt
- 1 tablespoon olive oil
- 2 cloves garlic, minced
- 2 tablespoons fresh parsley, chopped

Directions:
1. Preheat oven to 375°F.
2. Place halibut on a parchment-lined baking sheet. Sprinkle evenly with pepper and salt.
3. In a small bowl, combine olive oil, garlic, and parsley.
4. Spread garlic and parsley mixture over halibut fillets.
5. Bake for 15-20 minutes, or until halibut is cooked through.

Nutrition values: Calories: 153 kcal, Carbohydrates: 0.9 g, Protein: 24.8 g, Fat: 5.1 g, Saturated Fat: 0.8 g, Cholesterol: 51 mg, Sodium: 204 mg

Grilled Halibut with Mango Salsa

Preparation time: 10 minutes
Cooking time: 10 minutes
Servings: 4

Ingredients:
- 4 (6-ounce) halibut fillets
- 1/4 teaspoon freshly ground black pepper
- 1/4 teaspoon salt
- 1 tablespoon olive oil
- 1 mango, diced
- 1/2 red onion, diced
- 1/2 jalapeno, minced
- 1/4 cup fresh cilantro, chopped
- 1/4 cup lime juice

Directions:
1. Preheat grill to medium-high heat.
2. Place halibut on a greased baking sheet. Sprinkle evenly with pepper and salt.
3. Grill halibut for 5-7 minutes, or until cooked through.
4. In a medium bowl, combine mango, onion, jalapeno, cilantro, and lime juice.

5. Serve grilled halibut with mango salsa.

Nutrition values: Calories: 167 kcal, Carbohydrates: 9.7 g, Protein: 24.2 g, Fat: 5 g, Saturated Fat: 0.7 g, Cholesterol: 51 mg, Sodium: 197 mg

Baked Tilapia with Tomatoes and Olives

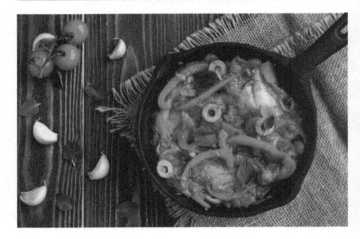

Preparation time: 10 minutes
Cooking time: 20 minutes
Servings: 4

Ingredients:
- 4 (6-ounce) tilapia fillets
- 1/4 teaspoon freshly ground black pepper
- 1/4 teaspoon salt
- 1 tablespoon olive oil
- 1 cup cherry tomatoes, halved
- 1/2 cup black olives, sliced
- 1/4 cup fresh parsley, chopped

Directions:
1. Preheat oven to 375°F.
2. Place tilapia on a parchment-lined baking sheet. Sprinkle evenly with pepper and salt.
3. Drizzle olive oil over tilapia.
4. Top with tomatoes and olives.

5. Bake for 15-20 minutes, or until tilapia is cooked through.
6. Sprinkle with parsley and serve.

Nutrition values: Calories: 169 kcal, Carbohydrates: 4.3 g, Protein: 25.4 g, Fat: 5.7 g, Saturated Fat: 0.8 g, Cholesterol: 51 mg, Sodium: 370 mg

Poached Cod with Lemon-Caper Sauce

Preparation time: 10 minutes
Cooking time: 10 minutes
Servings: 4

Ingredients:
*   4 (6-ounce) cod fillets
*   1/4 teaspoon freshly ground black pepper
*   1/4 teaspoon salt
*   1 tablespoon olive oil
*   1/4 cup white wine
*   1/4 cup lemon juice
*   2 tablespoons capers, drained
*   2 cloves garlic, minced
*   1/4 cup fresh parsley, chopped

Directions:
1. Place cod fillets in a large saucepan. Sprinkle evenly with pepper and salt.
2. Pour in wine, lemon juice, and enough water to cover the fish.
3. Bring to a boil, then reduce heat and simmer for 8-10 minutes, or until cod is cooked through.
4. In a small bowl, combine capers, garlic, and parsley.
5. Serve cod with lemon-caper sauce.

Nutrition values: Calories: 150 kcal, Carbohydrates: 2.3 g, Protein: 24.2 g, Fat: 4.4 g, Saturated Fat: 0.6 g, Cholesterol: 51 mg, Sodium: 375 mg

Broiled Cod with Mango Salsa

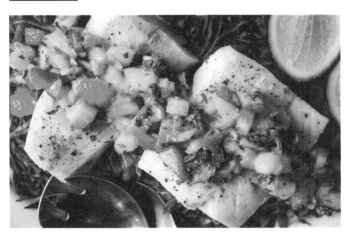

Preparation time: 10 minutes
Cooking time: 10 minutes
Servings: 2

Ingredients:
*   2 (6-ounce) cod fillets
*   1 tablespoon extra-virgin olive oil
*   ¼ teaspoon paprika
*   ¼ teaspoon garlic powder
*   Salt and fresh ground pepper to taste
*   ½ cup diced mango
*   ¼ cup diced red onion
*   1 tablespoon chopped fresh cilantro
*   1 tablespoon freshly squeezed lime juice

Directions:
1. Preheat broiler to high heat.
2. Place cod fillets on a baking sheet. Drizzle with olive oil, and season with paprika, garlic powder, salt, and pepper.
3. Broil for 5 minutes.
4. Meanwhile, in a bowl, combine mango, red onion, cilantro, and lime juice.
5. Flip cod fillets, and broil for an additional 5 minutes.
6. Serve cod with mango salsa.

Nutrition values: Calories: 229, Fat: 7.3g, Carbohydrates: 9.7g, Protein: 29.1g

Baked Trout with Herbs and Lemon

Preparation time: 10 minutes
Cooking time: 25 minutes
Servings: 2

Ingredients:
- 2 (6-ounce) trout fillets
- 2 tablespoons freshly squeezed lemon juice
- 1 tablespoons minced garlic
- 2 tablespoons capers
- 2 tablespoons extra-virgin olive oil
- 2 tablespoons chopped fresh parsley
- 1 tablespoons chopped fresh thyme
- Salt and fresh ground pepper to taste

Directions:
1. Preheat oven to 400 degrees F.
2. Place trout fillets in a greased baking dish.
3. In a bowl, mix together lemon juice, garlic, capers, olive oil, parsley, thyme, salt, and pepper.
4. Pour the mixture over the trout fillets.
5. Bake for 25 minutes, or until the trout flakes easily with a fork.

Nutrition values: Calories: 319, Fat: 16.2g, Carbohydrates: 1.6g, Protein: 38.7g

Grilled Trout with Mushrooms and Lemon

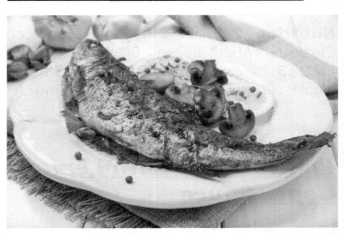

Preparation time: 10 minutes
Cooking time: 10 minutes
Servings: 2

Ingredients:
- 2 (6-ounce) trout fillets
- 2 tablespoons extra-virgin olive oil
- 1 tablespoon freshly squeezed lemon juice
- 1 tablespoon minced garlic
- ½ cup sliced mushrooms
- Salt and fresh ground pepper to taste

Directions:
1. Preheat a grill to medium-high heat.
2. Brush trout fillets with olive oil, and season with lemon juice, garlic, salt, and pepper.
3. Place trout fillets and mushrooms on the grill.
4. Grill for 5 minutes.
5. Flip trout fillets and mushrooms, and grill for an additional 5 minutes.

Nutrition values: Calories: 276, Fat: 16.1g, Carbohydrates: 1.5g, Protein: 32.2g

Mediterranean-Style Baked Salmon

Preparation time: 10 minutes
Cooking time: 20 minutes
Servings: 2
Ingredients:
- 2 (6-ounce) salmon fillets
- 1 tablespoon extra-virgin olive oil
- 2 tablespoons lemon juice
- 1 tablespoon minced garlic
- 2 tablespoons capers
- 2 tablespoons fresh oregano
- 2 tablespoons chopped fresh basil
- Salt and ground pepper to taste

Directions:
1. Preheat oven to 375 degrees F.
2. Place salmon fillets in a greased baking dish.
3. Drizzle with olive oil, and season with lemon juice, garlic, capers, oregano, basil, salt, and pepper.
4. Roast for 20 minutes, or until the salmon flakes easily.

Nutrition values: Calories: 294, Fat: 15.7g, Carbohydrates: 1.7g, Protein: 35.7g

Cajun-Style Baked Red Snapper

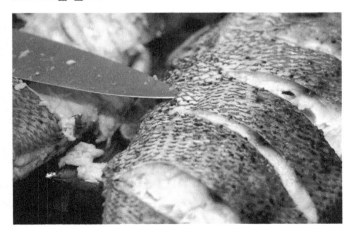

Preparation time: 10 minutes

Cooking time: 20 minutes
Servings: 4

Ingredients:
- 4 (6-ounce) red snapper fillets
- 1 tablespoon olive oil
- 2 tablespoons Cajun seasoning
- 2 tablespoons freshly squeezed lemon juice
- 2 tablespoons chopped fresh parsley
- 1 teaspoon freshly ground black pepper

Directions:
1. Preheat oven to 400°F.
2. Place the snapper fillets on a greased baking sheet.
3. Drizzle the olive oil over the fillets and sprinkle the Cajun seasoning, lemon juice, parsley, and pepper over the top.
4. Bake for 15 to 20 minutes, or until the fish is cooked through and flakes easily with a fork.

Nutrition Values: Calories: 180; Fat: 7g; Carbohydrates: 2g; Protein: 26g

Grilled Mackerel with Lemon-Garlic Butter

Preparation time: 10 minutes
Cooking time: 10 minutes
Servings: 4

Ingredients:
- 4 (4-ounce) mackerel fillets
- 1 tablespoon olive oil
- 1/4 teaspoon salt
- 1/4 teaspoon black pepper
- 2 tablespoons butter
- 2 cloves garlic, minced
- 2 tablespoons fresh lemon juice

Directions:
1. Preheat an outdoor grill or indoor grill pan to medium-high heat.

2. Brush mackerel fillets with olive oil and season with salt and pepper.
3. Place the fillets on the preheated grill and cook for 5 minutes per side or until cooked through.
4. In a small saucepan, melt butter over low heat. Add garlic and cook, stirring, for 1 minute.
5. Add lemon juice.
6. Drizzle garlic-lemon butter over cooked mackerel and serve.

Nutrition values: Calories: 153, Fat: 9g, Carbohydrates: 0g, Protein: 17g

Poached Mackerel with Ginger-Lime Sauce

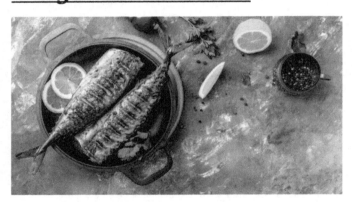

Preparation time: 15 minutes
Cooking time: 10 minutes
Servings: 4

Ingredients:
- 4 (4-ounce) mackerel fillets
- 1/4 teaspoon salt
- 1/4 teaspoon black pepper
- 1/2 cup chicken broth
- 2 tablespoons fresh lime juice
- 1 teaspoon grated fresh ginger
- 1/4 teaspoon red pepper flakes

Directions:
1. Place mackerel fillets in a large skillet and season with salt and pepper.
2. Add chicken broth to the skillet and bring to a boil.

3. Reduce heat to low, cover, and simmer for 10 minutes or until fish is cooked through.
4. In a small bowl, combine lime juice, ginger, and red pepper flakes.
5. Pour ginger-lime sauce over cooked mackerel and serve.

Nutrition values: Calories: 121, Fat: 5g, Carbohydrates: 1g, Protein: 17g

Baked Mahi-Mahi with Coconut-Lime Sauce

Preparation time: 10 minutes
Cooking time: 20 minutes
Servings: 4

Ingredients:
- 4 (6-ounce) mahi-mahi fillets
- 2 tablespoons olive oil
- 1/4 teaspoon salt
- 1/4 teaspoon black pepper
- 1/2 cup coconut milk
- 2 tablespoons fresh lime juice
- 1 teaspoon grated fresh ginger
- 1/4 teaspoon red pepper flakes

Directions:
1. Preheat oven to 375°F.
2. Place mahi-mahi fillets in a shallow baking dish.
3. Drizzle with olive oil and season with salt and pepper.
4. Bake in preheated oven for 20 minutes or until fish is cooked through and flakes easily with a fork.
5. Meanwhile, in a small saucepan, heat coconut milk over medium heat.
6. Add lime juice, ginger, and red pepper flakes. Simmer for 5 minutes.
7. Drizzle coconut-lime sauce over cooked mahi-mahi and serve.

Nutrition values: Calories: 191, Fat: 8g, Carbohydrates: 3g, Protein: 25g

Mahi-Mahi with Pineapple Salsa

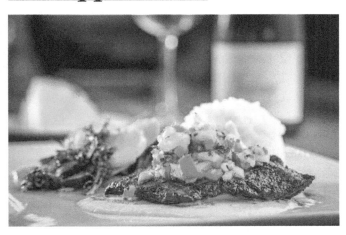

Preparation Time: 10 minutes
Cooking Time: 10 minutes
Servings: 4

Ingredients:
- 4 (6-ounce) mahi-mahi fillets
- 2 tablespoons olive oil
- 1/2 teaspoon salt
- 1/4 teaspoon black pepper
- 1 cup diced fresh pineapple
- 1/4 cup diced red onion
- 1 jalapeno, seeded and minced
- 2 tablespoons chopped fresh cilantro
- 2 teaspoons lime juice

Directions:
1. Heat the oil in a large skillet over medium-high heat.
2. Sprinkle the mahi-mahi with salt and pepper. Place the fish in the skillet and cook until golden and cooked through, about 3 minutes per side.
3. Meanwhile, in a medium bowl, combine the pineapple, red onion, jalapeno, cilantro, and lime juice.
4. Serve the fish with the pineapple salsa.

Baked Flounder with Mushrooms and Parmesan

Preparation Time: 10 minutes
Cooking Time: 30 minutes
Servings: 4

Ingredients:
- 4 (6-ounce) flounder fillets
- 1 teaspoon olive oil
- 1/2 teaspoon salt
- 1/4 teaspoon black pepper
- 1 cup sliced fresh mushrooms
- 1/4 cup grated Parmesan cheese

Directions:
1. Preheat the oven to 375 degrees F.
2. Grease a baking dish with the olive oil.
3. Place the flounder fillets in the baking dish and season with salt and pepper.
4. Top with the mushrooms and Parmesan cheese.
5. Bake for 20 to 25 minutes, or until the fish is cooked through and the cheese is melted and golden.

Nutrition Values: Calories: 189; Fat: 8.6g; Carbohydrates: 2.1g; Protein: 24.0g

Grilled Barramundi with Tomato-Basil Relish

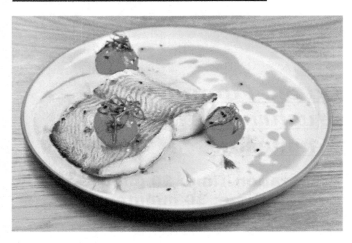

Preparation Time: 10 minutes
Cooking Time: 12 minutes
Servings: 4

Ingredients:
- 4 (6-ounce) barramundi fillets
- 2 tablespoons olive oil
- 1/2 teaspoon salt
- 1/4 teaspoon black pepper
- 1/2 cup diced tomatoes
- 1/4 cup chopped fresh basil
- 1 tablespoon lemon juice

Directions:
1. Heat a grill to medium-high heat.
2. Brush the barramundi fillets with the olive oil and season with salt and pepper.
3. Place the fillets on the grill and cook for 6 minutes per side, or until cooked through.
4. Meanwhile, in a small bowl, combine the tomatoes, basil, and lemon juice.
5. Serve the fillets with the tomato-basil relish.

Nutrition Values: Calories: 199; Fat: 9.4g; Carbohydrates: 0.9g; Protein: 25.1g

Grilled Sardines

Preparation Time: 5 minutes
Cooking Time: 8 minutes
Servings: 4

Ingredients:
- 4 sardines, cleaned and boned
- 2 tablespoons olive oil
- 1/2 teaspoon salt
- 1/4 teaspoon black pepper

Directions:
1. Heat a grill to medium-high heat.
2. Brush the sardines with the olive oil and season with salt and pepper.
3. Place the sardines on the grill and cook for 4 minutes per side, or until cooked through.
4. Serve the sardines hot off the grill.

Nutrition Values: Calories: 127; Fat: 7.2g; Carbohydrates: 0.0g; Protein: 15.6g

VEGETARIAN AND VEGAN RECIPES

Mediterranean Quinoa Bowl

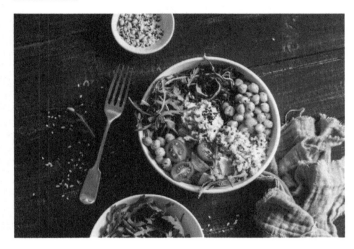

Preparation Time: 10 minutes
Cooking Time: 30 minutes
Servings: 4

Ingredients:
- 2 cups vegetable broth
- 1 cup quinoa
- 1 cup cherry tomatoes, halved
- 1/2 cup diced red onion
- 1/4 cup diced cucumber
- 1/4 cup pitted kalamata olives
- 2 tablespoons olive oil
- 2 tablespoons chopped fresh basil
- 2 tablespoons balsamic vinegar
- 1/4 teaspoon sea salt
- 1/4 teaspoon black pepper

Directions:
1. Bring the vegetable broth to a boil in a saucepan over high heat.
2. Add the quinoa, reduce the heat to low, and simmer for 20 minutes or until the quinoa is tender.
3. Remove the pan from the heat and set aside to cool.
4. In a large bowl, combine the cooked quinoa, tomatoes, onion, cucumber, olives, olive oil, basil, vinegar, salt, and pepper.
5. Toss to combine.
6. Serve the quinoa bowl warm or cold.

Nutrition Values: Calories: 330; Fat: 15g; Carbohydrates: 37g; Protein: 8g

Lentil Stew

Preparation Time: 10 minutes
Cooking Time: 30 minutes
Servings: 4

Ingredients:
- 1 tablespoon olive oil
- 1 large onion, diced
- 2 cloves garlic, minced
- 1 large carrot, chopped
- 2 stalks celery, chopped
- 2 cups vegetable broth
- 1 cup dried green lentils
- 1 teaspoon dried thyme
- 1/2 teaspoon dried oregano
- 1/4 teaspoon sea salt
- 1/4 teaspoon black pepper

Directions:
1. Heat the olive oil in a large saucepan over medium heat.
2. Add the onion and garlic and cook until tender, about 5 minutes.
3. Add the carrot and celery and cook for another 3 minutes.
4. Add the vegetable broth, lentils, thyme, oregano, salt, and pepper and bring to a boil.
5. Reduce the heat to low and simmer for 20 minutes or until the lentils are tender.
6. Serve the stew warm.

Nutrition Values: Calories: 250; Fat: 5g; Carbohydrates: 38g; Protein: 13g

Stuffed Peppers

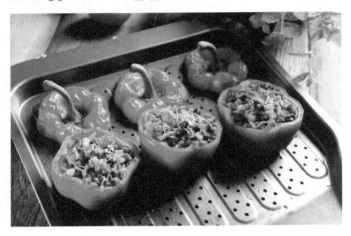

Preparation Time: 10 minutes
Cooking Time: 25 minutes
Servings: 4

Ingredients:
- 4 bell peppers, halved and seeded
- 1 tablespoon olive oil
- 1 large onion, diced
- 1 clove garlic, minced
- 1 cup cooked quinoa
- 1/2 cup cooked black beans
- 1/4 cup diced tomatoes
- 1 teaspoon ground cumin
- 1/4 teaspoon sea salt
- 1/4 teaspoon black pepper

Directions:
1. Preheat the oven to 375°F.
2. Place the bell pepper halves in a baking dish and set aside.
3. Fry the olive oil in a large pan over medium heat.
4. Add the onion and garlic and cook until tender, about 5 minutes.
5. Add the quinoa, black beans, tomatoes, cumin, salt, and pepper and cook for another 5 minutes.
6. Stuff the bell pepper halves with the quinoa mixture.
7. Bake for 20 minutes or until the peppers are tender.

Nutrition Values: Calories: 220; Fat: 5g; Carbohydrates: 33g; Protein: 9g

Roasted Veggie Wraps

Preparation Time: 10 minutes
Cooking Time: 25 minutes
Servings: 4
Ingredients:
- 2 zucchinis, sliced
- 2 red bell peppers, sliced
- 2 tablespoons olive oil
- 1/2 teaspoon sea salt
- 1/4 teaspoon black pepper
- 4 whole wheat tortillas
- 1/4 cup hummus
- 1/4 cup feta cheese, crumbled

Directions:
1. Preheat the oven to 375°F.
2. Place the zucchini and bell peppers in a large bowl and toss with the olive oil, salt, and pepper.
3. Spread the vegetables on a baking sheet and roast for 20 minutes or until tender.
4. Heat the tortillas in a skillet over medium heat for 1 minute on each side.
5. Spread the hummus on the tortillas and top with the roasted vegetables and feta cheese.
6. Roll the tortillas and serve.

Nutrition Values: Calories: 280; Fat: 14g; Carbohydrates: 31g; Protein: 8g

Sweet Potato and Black Bean Tacos

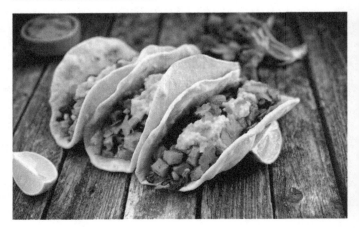

Preparation time: 10 minutes
Cooking time: 20 minutes
Servings: 4 tacos

Ingredients:
- 2 large sweet potatoes, cut into cubes
- 1 tablespoon olive oil
- 1/2 teaspoon ground cumin
- 1/2 teaspoon chili powder
- 1/2 teaspoon garlic powder
- 1/4 teaspoon salt
- 1 (15-ounce) can black beans, rinsed and drained
- 4 (6-inch) whole wheat tortillas
- 1/2 cup shredded lettuce
- 2 tablespoons chopped fresh cilantro
- 2 tablespoons diced red onion

Directions:
1. Preheat oven to 425°F.
2. Place sweet potatoes on a large baking sheet and toss with olive oil, cumin, chili powder, garlic powder, and salt.
3. Bake for 20 minutes or until potatoes are tender, stirring once halfway through.
4. Heat black beans in a small saucepan over medium heat for about 5 minutes.
3. Divide sweet potatoes and beans among the tortillas and top with lettuce, cilantro, and red onion.
4. Serve warm.

Nutrition values: Calories: 290, Fat: 6 g, Carbohydrates: 45 g, Protein: 11 g

Kale and White Bean Soup

Preparation time: 10 minutes
Cooking time: 30 minutes
Servings: 4

Ingredients:
- 1 tablespoon olive oil
- 1 onion, diced
- 4 cloves garlic, minced
- 4 cups vegetable broth
- 2 teaspoons dried oregano
- 2 teaspoons dried basil
- 1/2 teaspoon ground black pepper
- 1 (15-ounce) can white beans, rinsed and drained
- 4 cups kale, chopped
- 1/4 cup freshly squeezed lemon juice

Directions:
1. Heat olive oil in a large pot over medium heat.
2. Add onion and garlic and cook for 5 minutes or until vegetables are softened.
3. Add vegetable broth, oregano, basil, and pepper and bring to a boil.
4. Reduce heat to low and stir in white beans and kale.
5. Simmer for 20 minutes or until vegetables are tender.
6. Stir in lemon juice and season with additional salt and pepper, if desired.
7. Serve warm.

Nutrition values: Calories: 272, Fat: 5 g, Carbohydrates: 42 g, Protein: 14 g

Avocado Toast

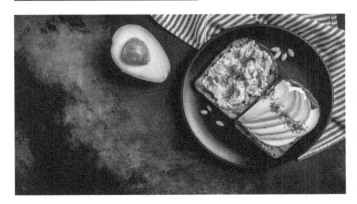

Preparation time: 5 minutes

Cooking time: 0 minutes
Servings: 1

Ingredients:
- 1 slice whole wheat bread
- 1/2 avocado, sliced
- 2 teaspoons olive oil
- 1/4 teaspoon garlic powder
- 1/4 teaspoon smoked paprika
- Salt and black pepper, to taste

Directions:
1. Toast the whole wheat bread in a toaster.
2. Top toast with avocado slices.
3. Drizzle with olive oil.
4. Sprinkle with garlic powder, smoked paprika, and season with salt and pepper.
5. Serve warm.

Nutrition values: Calories: 279, Fat: 15 g, Carbohydrates: 30 g, Protein: 5 g

Coconut Curry

Preparation time: 10 minutes
Cooking time: 30 minutes
Servings: 4

Ingredients:
- 2 tablespoons coconut oil
- 1 onion, diced
- 2 cloves garlic, minced
- 2 tablespoons fresh ginger, grated
- 1 tablespoon curry powder
- 1 teaspoon ground turmeric
- 1 teaspoon ground coriander
- 1/4 teaspoon ground cumin
- 1 (14-ounce) can light coconut milk
- 2 cups vegetable broth
- 1 head cauliflower, cut into florets
- 1 (15-ounce) can chickpeas, rinsed and drained
- 2 cups baby spinach
- Salt and black pepper, to taste

Directions:
1. Heat coconut oil in a large pot over medium heat.
2. Add onion, garlic, and ginger and cook for 5 minutes, or until vegetables are softened.
3. Add curry powder, turmeric, coriander, and cumin and cook for 1 minute.
4. Pour in coconut milk and vegetable broth and bring to a boil.
5. Add cauliflower, reduce heat to low, and simmer for 20 minutes.
6. Add chickpeas and spinach and simmer for an additional 5 minutes.
7. Season with salt and pepper, if desired.
8. Serve warm.

Nutrition values: Calories: 295, Fat: 15 g, Carbohydrates: 35 g, Protein: 9 g

Grilled Vegetable Skewers

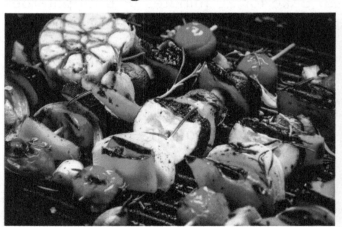

Preparation Time: 15 minutes
Cooking Time: 15 minutes
Servings: 4

Ingredients:
- 1 red bell pepper, cut into 2-inch pieces
- 1 yellow bell pepper, cut into 2-inch pieces
- 1 zucchini, cut into 2-inch pieces

- 1 red onion, cut into 2-inch pieces
- 1/4 cup extra-virgin olive oil
- 1 teaspoon Italian seasoning
- 1/2 teaspoon garlic powder
- 1/2 teaspoon sea salt

Directions:
1. Preheat the grill to medium heat.
2. In a medium-large bowl, combine the bell peppers, zucchini, and red onion.
3. Drizzle the vegetables with olive oil, Italian seasoning, garlic powder, and sea salt. Toss until the vegetables are evenly coated.
4. Thread the vegetables onto metal or wooden skewers.
5. Place the skewers on the preheated grill and cook for 8-10 minutes, turning halfway through.
6. Serve warm.

Nutrition Values: Calories: 151, Fat: 11.8g, Carbohydrates: 8.3g, Protein: 2.7g

Falafel Platter

Preparation Time: 20 minutes
Cooking Time: 15 minutes
Servings: 4

Ingredients:
- 1 cup dry chickpeas, soaked overnight
- 1/2 cup fresh parsley
- 1/4 cup fresh cilantro
- 1/4 cup diced red onion
- 2 cloves garlic, minced
- 2 tablespoons tahini
- 1 teaspoon ground cumin
- 1/4 teaspoon sea salt
- 1/4 teaspoon black pepper
- 3 tablespoons olive oil

Directions:
1. Drain and rinse the chickpeas, then place them in a food processor.

2. Add the parsley, cilantro, red onion, garlic, tahini, cumin, salt, and pepper. Pulse until the ingredients are combined and the mixture is crumbly.
3. Scoop the mixture out of the food processor and form it into 4-inch patties.
4. Fry the olive oil in a large pan over medium heat.
5. Place the patties in the skillet and cook for 7-8 minutes, flipping once.
6. Serve with a side of tahini, hummus, or other desired condiments.

Nutrition Values: Calories: 252, Fat: 15.3g, Carbohydrates: 23.2g, Protein: 6.3g

Vegetarian Chili

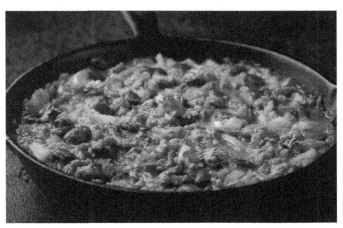

Preparation Time: 10 minutes
Cooking Time: 30 minutes
Servings: 4

Ingredients:
- 1 tablespoon olive oil
- 1 small onion, diced
- 2 cloves garlic, minced
- 1 red bell pepper, diced
- 1 zucchini, diced
- 1 (14-ounce) can diced tomatoes
- 1 (15-ounce) can black beans, drained and rinsed
- 1 (15-ounce) can kidney beans, drained and rinsed

- 1 cup vegetable broth
- 2 tablespoons chili powder
- 1 teaspoon ground cumin
- 1/2 teaspoon dried oregano
- 1/2 teaspoon sea salt
- 1/4 teaspoon black pepper

Directions:
1. Heat the olive oil in a large pot over medium heat.
2. Add the onion, garlic, bell pepper, and zucchini. Cook for 5 minutes, stirring occasionally.
3. Add the diced tomatoes, black beans, kidney beans, vegetable broth, chili powder, cumin, oregano, salt, and pepper. Stir to combine.
4. Increase the heat to high and bring the mixture to a boil.
5. Reduce the heat to low and simmer for 20-25 minutes, stirring occasionally.
6. Serve warm.

Nutrition Values: Calories: 280, Fat: 3.7g, Carbohydrates: 50.7g, Protein: 12.1g

Tomato Basil Frittata

Preparation Time: 10 minutes
Cooking Time: 15 minutes
Servings: 4

Ingredients:
- 1 tablespoon olive oil
- 1 small onion, diced
- 2 cloves garlic, minced
- 1 cup cherry tomatoes, halved
- 3 large eggs
- 1/4 cup milk
- 1/2 cup shredded mozzarella cheese
- 2 tablespoons chopped fresh basil
- 1/4 teaspoon sea salt
- 1/4 teaspoon black pepper

Directions:

1. Fry the olive oil in a large pan over medium heat.
2. Add the onion and garlic and cook for 3-4 minutes, stirring occasionally.
3. Add the cherry tomatoes and cook for another 2 minutes.
4. In a medium bowl, whisk the eggs, milk, mozzarella cheese, basil, salt, and pepper.
5. Pour the egg mixture into the skillet and cook for 5-7 minutes, until the eggs are set.
6. Serve warm.

Nutrition Values: Calories: 174, Fat: 11.3g, Carbohydrates: 6.3g, Protein: 11.1g

Portobello Burgers

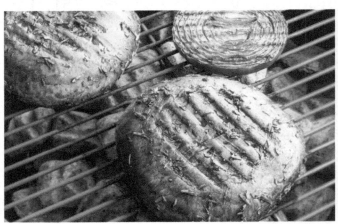

Preparation time: 10 minutes
Cooking time: 10 minutes
Servings: 4

Ingredients:
- 4 large Portobello mushrooms, stemmed and gills removed
- 1/4 cup olive oil
- 2 cloves garlic, minced
- 2 tablespoons balsamic vinegar
- 1 teaspoon dried oregano
- 1/2 teaspoon dried thyme
- 1/2 teaspoon sea salt
- 1/4 teaspoon freshly ground black pepper

- 4 whole-wheat hamburger buns

Directions:
1. Preheat the oven to 375 degrees F.
2. In a large bowl, combine the mushrooms, oil, garlic, balsamic vinegar, oregano, thyme, salt, and pepper. Toss to combine.
3. Place the mushrooms on a baking sheet and roast in the preheated oven for 8-10 minutes, flipping once halfway through.
4. Toast the buns in the oven for the last few minutes of roasting.
5. Serve the Portobello Burgers on toasted buns.

Nutrition values: Calories: 186, Fat: 11g, Carbohydrates: 16g, Protein: 7g

Eggplant Parmesan

Preparation time: 10 minutes
Cooking time: 40 minutes
Servings: 6

Ingredients:
- 1 large eggplant, cut into ½-inch slices
- ½ cup whole-wheat breadcrumbs
- 1/4 cup freshly grated Parmesan cheese
- 1 teaspoon dried oregano
- 1/2 teaspoon dried basil
- 1/4 teaspoon garlic powder
- 1/4 teaspoon sea salt
- 2 tablespoons olive oil
- 1/2 cup marinara sauce
- 1/2 cup shredded mozzarella cheese

Directions:
1. Preheat oven to 375 degrees F.
2. In a shallow bowl, combine the breadcrumbs, Parmesan cheese, oregano, basil, garlic powder, and salt.

3. Dip each eggplant slice in the breadcrumb mixture, coating both sides.
4. Heat the olive oil in a large skillet over medium-high heat.
5. Working in batches, cook the eggplant slices in the hot oil until golden brown, about 3 minutes per side.
6. Place the eggplant slices in a 9x13 inch baking dish.
7. Cover the eggplant slices with marinara sauce and top with mozzarella cheese.
8. Bake in preheated oven for 25-30 minutes, or until cheese is melted and bubbly.

Nutrition values: Calories: 166, Fat: 9g, Carbohydrates: 13g, Protein: 8g

Mediterranean Pasta Salad

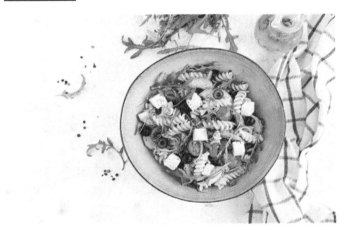

Preparation time: 10 minutes
Cooking time: 20 minutes
Servings: 4

Ingredients:
- 2 cups cooked whole grain or gluten-free pasta
- 2 cups chopped fresh tomatoes
- 1/2 cup chopped fresh basil
- 1/2 cup chopped red onion
- 1/2 cup sliced black olives
- 1/4 cup extra-virgin olive oil

- 4 tablespoons balsamic vinegar
- Salt and pepper to taste

Directions:
1. Cook the pasta following to package directions.
2. In a large bowl, combine the cooked pasta, tomatoes, basil, onion, and olives.
3. In a small bowl, whisk together the olive oil and vinegar.
4. Pour the dressing over the pasta salad and mix to combine.
5. Add salt and pepper to taste.
6. Serve chilled or at room temperature.

Nutrition values: Calories: 294; Fat: 16.2g; Carbohydrates: 29.3g; Protein: 6.2g

Roasted Ratatouille

Preparation time: 10 minutes
Cooking time: 40 minutes
Servings: 4

Ingredients:
- 2 tablespoons olive oil
- 1 large onion, diced
- 2 cloves garlic, minced
- 1 red bell pepper, diced
- 1 yellow bell pepper, diced
- 1 large eggplant, diced
- 2 large zucchini, diced
- 1 28-ounce can diced tomatoes
- 1 teaspoon dried oregano
- 1/2 teaspoon dried basil
- 1/2 teaspoon sea salt
- 1/4 teaspoon freshly ground black pepper

Directions:
1. Preheat oven to 375 degrees F.
2. Heat the olive oil in a large skillet over medium heat. Add the onion and garlic and cook about 4-5 minutes.

3. Add the bell peppers, eggplant, and zucchini and cook for another 5 minutes.
4. Pour the mixture into a 9x13 inch baking dish.
5. Pour the diced tomatoes over the vegetables and sprinkle with oregano, basil, salt, and pepper.
6. Cover the dish with aluminum foil and bake in preheated oven for 25-30 minutes, or until vegetables are tender.

Nutrition values: Calories: 201, Fat: 7g, Carbohydrates: 33g, Protein: 6g

Spinach Artichoke Dip

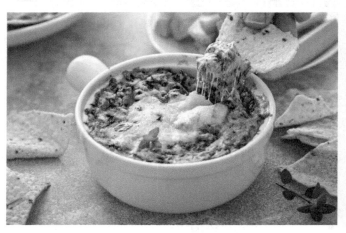

Preparation time: 10 minutes
Cooking time: 25 minutes
Servings: 8

Ingredients:
- 1 (10-ounce) package frozen chopped spinach, thawed and drained
- 1 (14-ounce) can artichoke hearts, drained and chopped
- 1/2 cup low-fat Greek yogurt
- 1/2 cup low-fat sour cream
- 1/3 cup finely grated Parmesan cheese
- 1/4 cup finely chopped onion
- 2 cloves garlic, minced
- 2 tablespoons freshly squeezed lemon juice
- 1/4 teaspoon red pepper flakes

- Salt and freshly ground black pepper

Directions:
1. Preheat oven to 375°F.
2. In a medium bowl, combine the spinach, artichoke hearts, yogurt, sour cream, Parmesan, onion, garlic, lemon juice, and red pepper flakes. Season with salt and pepper, to taste.
3. Transfer the mixture to a 9-inch pie plate or oven-safe dish and bake for 25 minutes, or until bubbling and golden brown.
4. Serve warm with toasted pita chips or crackers.

Nutrition values: Calories: 135; Fat: 4g; Carbohydrates: 13g; Protein: 8g

Zucchini Fritters

Preparation time: 10 minutes
Cooking time: 5 minutes
Servings: 4

Ingredients:
- 2 large zucchini, grated
- 1/4 cup all-purpose flour
- 1/2 teaspoon garlic powder
- 1/2 teaspoon onion powder
- 1/2 teaspoon dried basil
- Salt and freshly ground black pepper
- 2 tablespoons olive oil

Directions:
1. In a large bowl, combine the grated zucchini, flour, garlic powder, onion powder, basil, and salt and pepper, to taste. Mix until the ingredients are evenly distributed.
2. Heat the olive oil in a large skillet over medium-high heat.

3. Once the oil is hot, drop the zucchini mixture into the skillet in 2-inch rounds. Cook for 2-3 minutes per side, or until golden brown.
4. Remove from the skillet and serve warm with your favorite dipping sauce.

Nutrition values: Calories: 117; Fat: 6g; Carbohydrates: 12g; Protein: 2g

Vegetable Lasagna

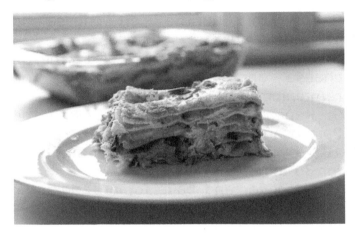

Preparation time: 15 minutes
Cooking time: 40 minutes
Servings: 8

Ingredients:
- 2 tablespoons olive oil
- 1 red bell pepper, diced
- 1 green bell pepper, diced
- 1 onion, diced
- 2 cloves garlic, minced
- 1 (14.5-ounce) can diced tomatoes, drained
- 2 (8-ounce) packages no-boil lasagna noodles
- 1 (15-ounce) container ricotta cheese
- 2 cups shredded mozzarella cheese
- 1/2 cup grated Parmesan cheese
- 2 tablespoons chopped fresh basil
- Salt and freshly ground black pepper

Directions:
1. Preheat oven to 375°F.
2. Heat the olive oil in a large skillet over medium-high heat.
3. Add the bell peppers, onion, and garlic and cook until softened, about 5 minutes.
4. Stir in the diced tomatoes and cook until heated through, about 2 minutes.
5. Spread 1/4 cup of the tomato mixture in the bottom of a 9x13-inch baking dish.
6. Place 2 layers of lasagna noodles on top of the tomato mixture.
7. Top with 1/2 of the ricotta cheese and 1/2 of the mozzarella cheese.
8. Sprinkle with 1/4 cup of Parmesan cheese and top with 1/2 of the remaining tomato mixture.
9. Repeat the layers, ending with the Parmesan cheese.
10. Cover the lasagna with foil and bake for 30 minutes.
11. Uncover and bake for an additional 10-15 minutes, or until the cheese is melted and lightly browned.
12. Let cool it for 10 minutes before serving.

Nutrition values: Calories: 284; Fat: 14g; Carbohydrates: 20g; Protein: 17g

- 2 tablespoons freshly squeezed lime juice
- 1/2 teaspoon red pepper flakes
- Salt and freshly ground black pepper

Directions:
1. Heat the sesame oil in a large skillet over medium-high heat.
2. Add the bell peppers, onion, and garlic and cook until softened, about 5 minutes.
3. Add the broccoli and cauliflower and cook until tender, about 5 minutes.
4. Stir in the soy sauce, lime juice, and red pepper flakes and season with salt and pepper, to taste.
5. Cook for an additional 2 minutes, or until the vegetables are cooked through.
6. Serve warm with steamed rice.

Nutrition values: (Per Serving)
Calories: 122; Fat: 6g; Carbohydrates: 13g; Protein: 5g

Vegetable Stir Fry

Preparation time: 10 minutes
Cooking time: 10 minutes
Servings: 4

Ingredients:
- 1 tablespoon sesame oil
- 1 red bell pepper, sliced
- 1 green bell pepper, sliced
- 1 onion, sliced
- 2 cloves garlic, minced
- 2 cups broccoli florets
- 2 cups cauliflower florets
- 1/4 cup low-sodium soy sauce

SNACKS RECIPES

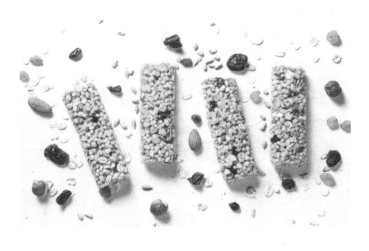

2. In the morning, stir in the chia seeds and berries. Enjoy!

Nutrition values: Calories: 242, Fat: 5.3g, Carbohydrates: 40.4g, Protein: 8.4g

Apple Slices with Almond Butter

Preparation time: 5 minutes
Cooking time: 0 minutes
Servings: 2

Ingredients:
- 2 apples, sliced
- 2 tablespoons almond butter
- 1 teaspoon ground cinnamon

Directions:
1. Slice the apples and spread each slice with a thin layer of almond butter. 2. Sprinkle with cinnamon and enjoy!

Nutrition values (2 servings): Calories: 215, Fat: 13.1g, Carbohydrates: 21.3g, Protein: 5.3g

Overnight Oats

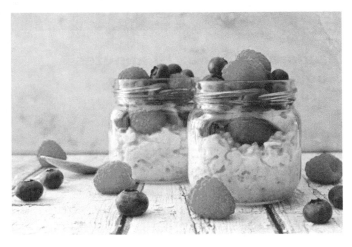

Preparation time: 10 minutes
Cooking time: 0 minutes
Servings: 1

Ingredients:
- ½ cup rolled oats
- ½ cup almond milk
- ½ teaspoon ground cinnamon
- ½ teaspoon honey
- 1 tablespoon chia seeds
- ½ cup fresh or frozen berries

Directions:
1. In a medium bowl, mix the oats, almond milk, cinnamon and honey. Cover and chill in the refrigerator overnight.

Trail Mix

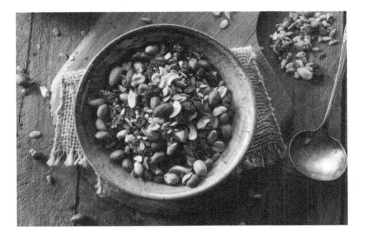

Preparation time: 10 minutes
Cooking time: 0 minutes

Servings: 10

Ingredients:
- 1/2 cup almonds
- 1/2 cup cashews
- 1/2 cup walnuts
- 1/2 cup dried cranberries
- 1/4 cup dark chocolate chips
- 1 tablespoon honey

Directions:
1. In a medium bowl, mix together all of the ingredients. Enjoy!

Nutrition values (per serving): Calories: 184, Fat: 11.9g, Carbohydrates: 14.2g, Protein: 5.4g

Sweet Potato Chips

Preparation time: 10 minutes
Cooking time: 30 minutes
Servings: 4

Ingredients:
- 2 sweet potatoes, sliced thinly
- 2 tablespoons olive oil
- 1 teaspoon ground cumin
- 1 teaspoon garlic powder
- 1/2 teaspoon sea salt

Directions:
1. Preheat oven to 375°F. Line a baking sheet with parchment paper.
2. In a small bowl, mix together the olive oil, cumin, garlic powder, and sea salt.
3. Arrange the sweet potato slices in a single layer on the prepared baking sheet. Brush the slices with the oil mixture and bake for 25-30 minutes, flipping halfway through, until golden brown and crispy.
4. Enjoy!

Nutrition values (1 serving): Calories: 154, Fat: 9.7g, Carbohydrates: 14.7g, Protein: 2.1g

Hummus with Veggies

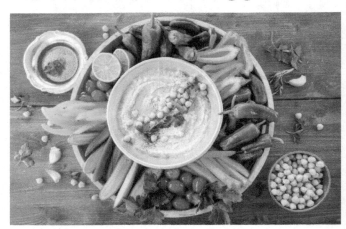

Preparation time: 10 minutes
Cooking time: 0 minutes
Servings: 2

Ingredients:
- 1 can of chickpeas
- 2 tablespoons of tahini
- 2 cloves of garlic, minced
- 2 tablespoons of freshly squeezed lemon juice
- 1/4 teaspoon of ground cumin
- 1/4 teaspoon of paprika
- 1/4 teaspoon of salt
- 1/4 cup of olive oil
- 2 cups of chopped vegetables (celery, carrots, bell peppers, cucumbers, etc.)

Directions:
1. Drain and rinse chickpeas in a colander and add to a food processor.
2. Add tahini, garlic, lemon juice, cumin, paprika, and salt.
3. Pulse the ingredients until they are combined.
4. Slowly add olive oil while the food processor is running and continue to blend until smooth.

5. Place the hummus in a bowl and serve with chopped vegetables.

Nutrition Values (per serving): Calories: 250; Fat: 17 g; Carbohydrates: 21 g; Protein: 8 g

Greek Yogurt

Preparation time: 5 minutes
Cooking time: 0 minutes
Servings: 1

Ingredients:
- 1 cup of plain Greek yogurt
- 1 teaspoon of honey
- 1/4 teaspoon of ground cinnamon
- 1/4 cup of fresh berries

Directions:
1. Place the Greek yogurt in a bowl.
2. Drizzle the honey and sprinkle the cinnamon over the yogurt.
3. Top with fresh berries.

Nutrition Values: Calories: 150; Fat: 5 g; Carbohydrates: 17 g; Protein: 10 g

Cucumber Slices with Cottage Cheese

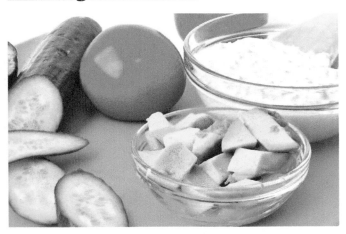

Preparation time: 5 minutes

Cooking time: 0 minutes
Servings: 1

Ingredients:
- 1 cup of cucumber slices
- 1/4 cup of cottage cheese
- 1/4 teaspoon of dill
- Salt and pepper to taste

Directions:
1. Place the cucumber slices on a plate.
2. Top with cottage cheese and sprinkle with dill, salt, and pepper.
3. Serve.

Nutrition Values: Calories: 70; Fat: 1g; Carbohydrates: 4g; Protein: 8g

Kale Chips

Preparation Time: 10 minutes
Cooking Time: 20 minutes
Servings: 4

Ingredients:
- 2 bunches of kale
- 2 tablespoons of olive oil
- 1 teaspoon of sea salt
- 1 teaspoon of garlic powder

Directions:
1. Preheat the oven to 375°F.
2. Wash and dry the kale. Remove the leaves from the stems and tear them into pieces.
3. Place the kale in a bowl and add the olive oil, salt, and garlic powder. Toss to combine.
4. Arrange the kale pieces on a baking sheet lined with parchment paper.
5. Bake for 15-20 minutes, or until the chips are crisp and lightly browned.
6. Serve immediately.

Nutrition Values (per serving): Calories: 80, Fat: 5g, Carbohydrates: 7g, Protein: 2g

Edamame

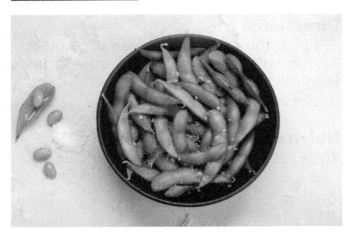

Preparation Time: 5 minutes
Cooking Time: 10 minutes
Servings: 4

Ingredients:
- 2 cups of edamame
- 2 teaspoons of olive oil
- 1 teaspoon of sea salt
- 1 teaspoon of garlic powder

Directions:
1. Bring a pot of salted water to a boil over high heat.
2. Add the edamame and cook for 5-7 minutes.
3. Drain the edamame and place in a bowl.
4. Add the olive oil, salt, and garlic powder. Toss to combine.
5. Serve immediately.

Nutrition Values (per serving): Calories: 80, Fat: 3.5g, Carbohydrates: 6g, Protein: 8g

Tuna Salad on Whole Wheat Crackers

Preparation Time: 10 minutes
Cooking Time: 0 minutes
Servings: 4

Ingredients:
- 2 cans of tuna, drained
- 2 tablespoons of mayonnaise
- 2 tablespoons of minced onion
- 1 teaspoon of lemon juice
- 1 teaspoon of Dijon mustard
- Salt and pepper to taste
- 1 package of whole wheat crackers

Directions:
1. In a medium bowl, combine the tuna, mayonnaise, onion, lemon juice, and mustard. Mix until well combined.
2. Season with salt and pepper to taste.
3. Spoon the tuna salad onto the crackers and serve.

Nutrition Values (per serving): Calories: 180, Fat: 8g, Carbohydrates: 18g, Protein: 12g

Chia Pudding

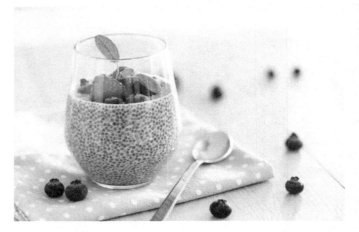

Preparation Time: 10 minutes
Cooking Time: 0 minutes

Servings: 4

Ingredients:
- 2 cups of almond milk
- ¼ cup of chia seeds
- 2 tablespoons of maple syrup
- 1 teaspoon of vanilla extract
- ½ teaspoon of ground cinnamon
- Toppings (optional): fresh fruit, chopped nuts, shredded coconut

Directions:
1. In a medium bowl, combine the almond milk, chia seeds, maple syrup, vanilla extract, and cinnamon. Stir until well combined.
2. Cover the bowl and refrigerate for at least 4 hours or overnight.
3. Serve chilled topped with desired toppings.

Nutrition Values (per serving): Calories: 160, Fat: 8g, Carbohydrates: 19g, Protein: 4g

Carrot Sticks with Hummus

Preparation time: 10 minutes
Cooking time: N/A
Servings: 2

Ingredients:
4 carrots, peeled and cut into sticks
4 tablespoons hummus

Directions:
1. Peel and cut the carrots into sticks.
2. Serve the carrots with hummus.

Nutrition values: Calories: 115, Fat: 5g, Carbohydrates: 14g, Protein: 3g.

Popcorn

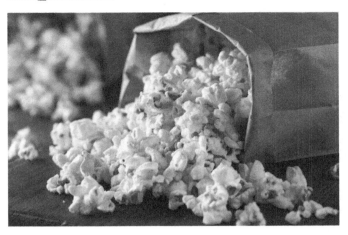

Preparation Time: 5 minutes
Cooking Time: 5 minutes
Servings: 4

Ingredients:
- 1/4 cup popcorn kernels
- 1 teaspoon olive oil
- Salt to taste

Directions:
1. Heat a medium-sized pot over medium heat.
2. When the pot is hot, add the olive oil and popcorn kernels.
3. Cover the pot with a lid and let the kernels pop, shaking the pot every few seconds.
4. Once the popping has stopped, remove the pot from the heat and pour the popcorn into a bowl.
5. Sprinkle with salt to taste and serve.

Nutrition values (per serving): Calories: 95; Fat: 5g; Carbohydrates: 11g; Protein: 2g

Smoothie Bowls

Preparation time: 10 minutes
Cooking time: N/A
Servings: 2

Ingredients:
- 1 banana, sliced
- 1 cup frozen berries
- ½ cup milk
- 2 tablespoons nut butter
- 2 tablespoons granola
- 2 tablespoons shredded coconut

Directions:
1. Place the banana, frozen berries, and milk in a blender and blend until smooth.
2. Pour the smoothie mixture into two bowls.
3. Top each smoothie bowl with nut butter, granola, and shredded coconut.

Nutrition values: Calories: 306, Fat: 14g, Carbohydrates: 37g, Protein: 9g.

Coconut Chips

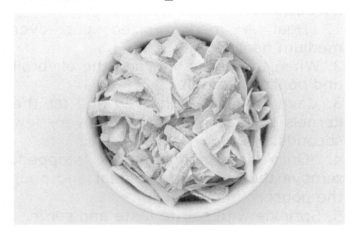

Preparation time: 10 minutes
Cooking time: 8 minutes
Servings: 4

Ingredients:
- 2 cups shredded coconut
- 1 tablespoon coconut oil
- 1 teaspoon salt
- 1 teaspoon sugar

Directions:
1. Preheat the oven to 350°F.

2. In a bowl, mix together the shredded coconut, coconut oil, salt, and sugar.
3. Spread the mixture onto a baking sheet lined with parchment paper.
4. Bake for 8 minutes, or until golden brown.
5. Let cool before serving.

Nutrition values: Calories: 170, Fat: 14g, Carbohydrates: 10g, Protein: 2g

Dark Chocolate

Preparation Time: 5 minutes
Cooking Time: 0 minutes
Servings: 1

Ingredients:
- 1 oz. dark chocolate (at least 70% cocoa)

Directions:
1. Break the chocolate bar into small pieces.
2. Place the pieces in a bowl.
3. Microwave the pieces for 30 seconds.
4. Stir until melted and smooth.

Nutrition values: Calories: 160, Fat: 11g, Carbohydrates: 15g, Protein: 2g

Quinoa Salad

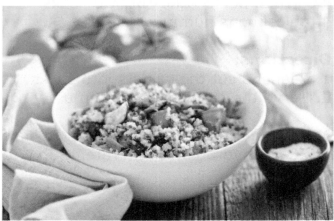

Preparation Time: 10 minutes

Cooking Time: 20 minutes
Servings: 4

Ingredients:
- 1 cup quinoa
- 2 cups of vegetable broth
- ½ cup of diced tomatoes
- ½ cup of diced red onion
- 2 tablespoons of olive oil
- 2 tablespoons of lemon juice
- 1 teaspoon of salt

Directions:
1. Rinse the quinoa in a strainer.
2. Place the quinoa and vegetable broth in a pot and bring to a boil.
3. Reduce the heat and let simmer for 20 minutes.
4. Transfer the quinoa to a large bowl and add the tomatoes, red onion, olive oil, lemon juice, and salt.
5. Mix until combined and serve.

Nutrition values (per serving): Calories: 242, Fat: 8g, Carbohydrates: 34g, Protein: 8g

Green Olives

Preparation Time: 5 minutes
Cooking Time: 0 minutes
Servings: 4

Ingredients:
- 1 cup of olives, pitted
- 2 tablespoons of olive oil
- 1 teaspoon of garlic, minced
- 1 teaspoon of lemon juice

Directions:
1. Place the olives in a bowl.
2. Drizzle the olive oil, garlic, and lemon juice over the olives and mix until all the olives are coated.
3. Serve and enjoy.

Nutrition values (per serving): Calories: 121, Fat: 11g, Carbohydrates: 4g, Protein: 1g

Berries with Almond Milk

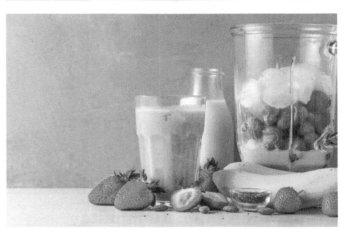

Preparation Time: 5 minutes
Cooking Time: 0 minutes
Servings: 1

Ingredients:
- 1 cup of frozen berries
- 1 cup of almond milk
- 1 tablespoon of honey

Directions:
1. Place the berries and almond milk in a blender.
2. Blend until smooth.
3. Add the honey and blend until incorporated.
4. Serve and enjoy.

Nutrition values: Calories: 190, Fat: 5g, Carbohydrates: 33g, Protein: 4g

DESSERT RECIPES

Sweet Potato Brownies

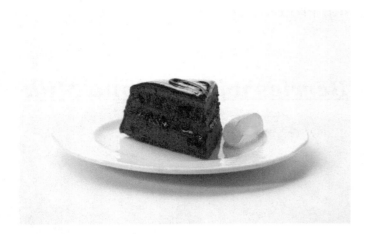

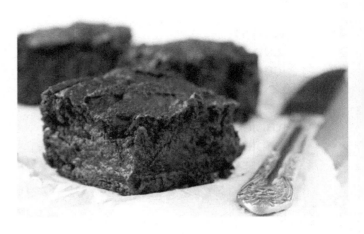

Preparation time: 15 minutes
Cooking time: 25 minutes
Servings: 16

Banana Date Walnut Bars

Preparation time: 10 minutes
Cooking time: 25 minutes
Servings: 15

Ingredients:
- 2 cups of mashed bananas
- 1 cup of dates, pitted and chopped
- 1 cup of walnuts, chopped
- 1/2 cup of almond flour
- 1/4 cup of coconut oil, melted
- 1/4 teaspoon of sea salt
- 1 teaspoon of ground cinnamon

Directions:
1. Preheat the oven to 350°F. Grease an 8×8 inch baking dish with coconut oil.
2. In a large bowl, mash the bananas until they are smooth.
3. Add the dates, walnuts, almond flour, coconut oil, sea salt and cinnamon. Stir until everything is well combined.
4. Pour the mixture into the baking dish. Spread it out evenly.
5. Bake for 25 minutes or until the top is golden brown.
6. Let cool before slicing into bars.

Nutrition values: Calories: 135; Fat: 8 g; Carbohydrates: 13 g; Protein: 2 g

Ingredients:
- 1 cup of mashed sweet potato
- 1/2 cup of almond butter
- 1/4 cup of maple syrup
- 1/4 cup of cocoa powder
- 1 teaspoon of vanilla extract
- 1/4 teaspoon of sea salt
- 1/2 cup of walnuts, chopped

Directions:
1. Preheat the oven to 340°F. Grease an 8×8 inch baking dish with coconut oil.
2. In a large bowl, mash the sweet potato until it is smooth.
3. Add the almond butter, maple syrup, cocoa powder, vanilla extract and sea salt. Stir until everything is well combined.
4. Fold in the walnuts.
5. Pour the mixture into the baking dish. Spread it out evenly.
6. Bake for 25 minutes or until the top is firm.
7. Let cool before slicing into bars.

Nutrition values: Calories: 145; Fat: 8g; Carbohydrates: 14g; Protein: 4g

Apple Crumble with Toasted Coconut

Preparation time: 15 minutes
Cooking time: 25 minutes
Servings: 8

Ingredients:
- 4 cups of apples, peeled and diced
- 1/4 cup of maple syrup
- 1/3 teaspoon of ground cinnamon
- 1/4 teaspoon of sea salt
- 1/2 cup of rolled oats
- 1/4 cup of almond flour
- 1/3 cup of coconut oil, melted
- 1/4 cup of shredded coconut, toasted

Directions:
1. Preheat the oven to 350°F. Grease an 8×8 inch baking dish with coconut oil.
2. In a large bowl, combine the apples, maple syrup, cinnamon and sea salt. Stir until everything is well combined.
3. Pour the mixture into the baking dish.
4. In a separate bowl, mix together the oats, almond flour, and coconut oil.
5. Sprinkle the topping over the apples.
6. Bake for 25 minutes or until the topping is golden brown.
7. Sprinkle with toasted coconut before serving.

Nutrition values (per serving): Calories: 160; Fat: 10g; Carbohydrates: 18g; Protein: 2g

Strawberry Rhubarb Crumble

Preparation time: 10 minutes
Cooking time: 25 minutes
Servings: 8

Ingredients:
- 2 cups of strawberries, sliced
- 2 cups of rhubarb, diced
- 1/4 cup of maple syrup
- 1/4 teaspoon of ground cinnamon
- 1/4 teaspoon of sea salt
- 1/2 cup of rolled oats
- 1/4 cup of almond flour
- 1/4 cup of coconut oil, melted
- 1/4 cup of walnuts, chopped

Directions:
1. Preheat the oven to 350°F. Grease an 8×8 inch baking dish with coconut oil.
2. In a large bowl, combine the strawberries, rhubarb, maple syrup, cinnamon and sea salt. Stir until everything is well combined.
3. Pour the mixture into the baking dish.
4. In a separate bowl, mix together the oats, almond flour, and coconut oil.
5. Sprinkle the topping over the fruit.
6. Bake for 25 minutes or until the topping is golden brown.
7. Sprinkle with walnuts before serving.

Nutrition values (per serving): Calories: 175; Fat: 11g; Carbohydrates: 18g; Protein: 3g

Baked Apples with Cinnamon and Maple Syrup

Preparation time: 10 minutes
Cooking time: 20 minutes
Servings: 4

Ingredients:
- 4 medium apples, peeled and cored
- 1/4 cup maple syrup
- 2 teaspoons ground cinnamon

Directions:
1. Preheat oven to 375°F.
2. Place the apples in a baking dish.

3. In a small bowl, mix together the maple syrup and cinnamon.
4. Pour the mixture over the apples and stir to coat.
5. Bake in the preheated oven for 20 minutes, or until the apples are tender.

Nutrition values: Calories: 144, Fat: 0.2g, Carbohydrates: 38g, Protein: 0.5g

Coconut Flour Carrot Cake

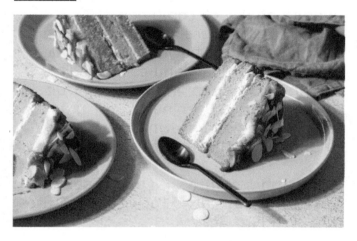

Preparation time: 10 minutes
Cooking time: 30 minutes
Servings: 12

Ingredients:
- 2 cups coconut flour
- 2 teaspoons baking powder
- 2 teaspoons ground cinnamon
- 1/2 teaspoon ground nutmeg
- 1/2 teaspoon salt
- 1/2 cup coconut oil, melted
- 1 cup maple syrup
- 4 eggs
- 2 teaspoons vanilla extract
- 2 cups grated carrots

Directions:
1. Preheat oven to 350°F.
2. In a large bowl, mix together the coconut flour, baking powder, cinnamon, nutmeg and salt.

3. In a separate bowl, whisk together the coconut oil, maple syrup, eggs, and vanilla extract.
4. Add the wet ingredients to the dry ingredients and mix until combined.
5. Stir in the grated carrots.
6. Grease a 9x13 inch baking dish with coconut oil.
7. Pour the batter into the prepared dish and spread evenly.
8. Bake in preheated oven for 30 minutes, or until a toothpick inserted into the center comes out clean.

Nutrition values: Calories: 254, Fat: 14.9g, Carbohydrates: 28.6g, Protein: 4.1g

Blueberry Almond Flour Muffins

Preparation time: 10 minutes
Cooking time: 25 minutes
Servings: 10

Ingredients:
- 2 cups almond flour
- 2 teaspoons baking powder
- 1/4 teaspoon salt
- 1/4 cup coconut oil, melted
- 3 eggs
- 1/4 cup honey
- 1 teaspoon vanilla extract
- 1 cup fresh blueberries

Directions:
1. Preheat oven to 350°F.
2. In a medium bowl, mix together the almond flour, baking powder and salt.
3. In a separate bowl, whisk together the coconut oil, eggs, honey and vanilla extract.
4. Add the wet ingredients to the dry ingredients and mix until combined.
5. Fold in the blueberries.
6. Grease a muffin tin with coconut oil.

7. Split the mixture equally among the muffin cups.

8. Bake in preheated oven for 25 minutes, or until a toothpick inserted into the center comes out clean.

Nutrition values (per serving): Calories: 182, Fat: 13.2g, Carbohydrates: 13.7g, Protein: 5.9g

Chocolate Avocado Pudding

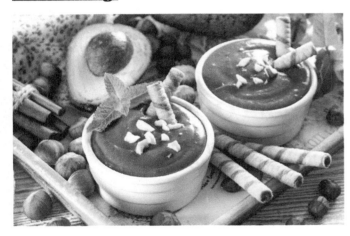

Preparation time: 10 minutes
Cooking time: 0 minutes
Servings: 4

Ingredients:
- 2 ripe avocados
- 1/4 cup cocoa powder
- 1/4 cup maple syrup
- 2 tablespoons coconut oil, melted
- 1 teaspoon vanilla extract

Directions:
1. In a food processor, mix the avocados.
2. Add the cocoa powder, maple syrup, coconut oil, and vanilla extract and blend until everything is well combined.
3. Divide the mixture evenly among four glasses.
4. Refrigerate for at least an hour before serving.

Nutrition values: Calories: 217, Fat: 15.2g, Carbohydrates: 21.2g, Protein: 3.3g

Almond Butter Brownies

Preparation time: 10 minutes
Cooking time: 30 minutes
Servings: 16

Ingredients:
- 1 cup almond butter
- 1/2 cup coconut sugar
- 1/4 cup maple syrup
- 1 teaspoon vanilla extract
- 1/3 cup cocoa powder
- 1 teaspoon baking soda
- 1/4 teaspoon salt
- 2 eggs

Directions:
1. Preheat oven to 350°F. Grease an 8×8 inch baking pan.
2. In a medium bowl, mix together almond butter, coconut sugar, maple syrup, and vanilla extract.
3. In a separate bowl, whisk together cocoa powder, baking soda, and salt.
4. Add the dry ingredients to the wet ingredients, and mix to combine.
5. Add eggs to the mixture, and mix until a thick batter forms.
6. Spread the mixture evenly into the prepared baking pan.
7. Bake for 25–30 minutes.
8. Allow to cool before slicing into 16 pieces.

Nutrition values (per serving): Calories: 187; Fat: 12.9g; Carbohydrates: 15.4g; Protein: 5.4g

Zucchini Cake with Lemon Glaze

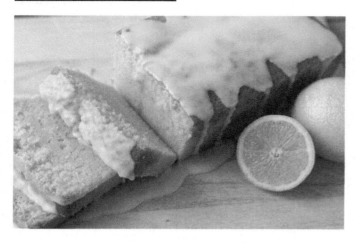

Preparation time: 15 minutes
Cooking time: 25 minutes
Servings: 12

Ingredients:
*   1 cup whole wheat flour
*   1 teaspoon baking soda
*   1/2 teaspoon baking powder
*   1/2 teaspoon salt
*   1 teaspoon ground cinnamon
*   1/4 teaspoon ground nutmeg
*   1/2 cup olive oil
*   1/2 cup honey
*   2 eggs
*   1 teaspoon vanilla extract
*   1 1/2 cups grated zucchini
*   1/2 cup chopped walnuts
*   1/2 cup raisins

For the Lemon Glaze:
*   1/4 cup lemon juice
*   1 cup powdered sugar

Directions:
1. Preheat oven to 350°F. Grease a 9×13 inch baking pan.
2. In a medium bowl, whisk together flour, baking soda, baking powder, salt, cinnamon, and nutmeg.
3. In a separate bowl, mix together olive oil, honey, eggs, and vanilla extract.
4. Add the dry ingredients to the wet ingredients, and mix until combined.
5. Fold in zucchini, walnuts, and raisins.
6. Spread the mixture evenly into the prepared baking pan.
7. Bake for 20–25 minutes, or until a toothpick inserted into the center comes out clean.
8. Allow to cool before frosting with lemon glaze.

To make the Lemon Glaze:
1. In a bowl, whisk lemon juice and powdered sugar until smooth.
2. Drizzle over cooled cake.

Nutrition values (per serving):
Calories: 267; Fat: 11.9g; Carbohydrates: 36.2g; Protein: 4.1g

Banana Oat Blondies

Preparation time: 15 minutes
Cooking time: 25 minutes
Servings: 16

Ingredients:
*   ½ cups of oat flour
*   ½ cup of coconut sugar
*   2 ripe bananas, mashed
*   ¼ cup of coconut oil, melted
*   ½ teaspoon of vanilla extract
*   ¼ teaspoon of sea salt
*   2 tablespoons of ground flaxseed
*   1 teaspoon of cinnamon
*   ½ teaspoon of baking soda

Directions:
1. Preheat the oven to 350°F and line an 8x8 baking pan with parchment paper.
2. In a medium-sized bowl, whisk together the oat flour, coconut sugar, baking soda, sea salt, and cinnamon.
3. In a separate bowl, mix together the mashed bananas, melted coconut oil, vanilla extract, and ground flaxseed.
4. Add the wet ingredients to the dry ingredients and mix until combined.

5. Pour the mixture into the prepared baking pan and spread it out evenly.
6. Bake for 25 minutes, or until the top is golden brown.
7. Let cool before cutting into 16 bars.

Nutrition values (per serving): Calories: 95; Fat: 5g; Carbohydrates: 11g; Protein: 1.5g

Spiced Pear Galette

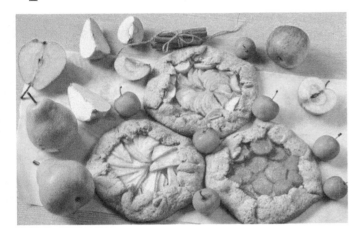

Preparation time: 10 minutes
Cooking time: 40 minutes
Servings: 8

Ingredients:
- 2 pears, sliced
- 1/4 cup brown sugar
- 1 teaspoon ground cinnamon
- 1/4 teaspoon ground nutmeg
- 1/4 teaspoon ground ginger
- 1/4 teaspoon ground allspice
- 1/4 teaspoon ground cloves
- 1/4 teaspoon salt
- 1/2 teaspoon lemon juice
- 1/4 cup almond flour
- 1/4 cup coconut oil, melted
- 1 teaspoon vanilla extract

Directions:
1. Preheat oven to 375°F. Grease an 8-inch round baking pan.

2. In a medium bowl, mix together pears, brown sugar, cinnamon, nutmeg, ginger, allspice, cloves, salt, and lemon juice.
3. In a separate bowl, whisk together almond flour, coconut oil, and vanilla extract.
4. Add the wet ingredients to the pear mixture, and mix to combine.
5. Spread the mixture evenly into the prepared baking pan.
6. Bake for 35–40 minutes, or until the edges are golden brown.
7. Allow to cool before slicing into 8 pieces.

Nutrition values (per serving): Calories: 172; Fat: 10.9g; Carbohydrates: 18.2g; Protein: 1.8g

Cocoa Almond Bites

Preparation time: 10 minutes
Cooking time: 10 minutes
Servings: 12

Ingredients:
- 2 tablespoons almond butter
- 1 tablespoon cocoa powder
- 2 tablespoons honey or maple syrup
- ¼ cup coconut flakes
- ¼ cup chopped almonds
- 2 tablespoons chia seeds

Directions:
1. Preheat oven to 350°F (175°C).
2. In a medium bowl, mix together almond butter, cocoa powder, honey or maple syrup, coconut flakes, chopped almonds, and chia seeds.
3. Line a baking sheet with parchment paper.
4. Form 12 small balls from the mixture and place on the baking sheet.
5. Bake for 10 minutes.
6. Let cool before serving.

Nutrition values: Calories: 84, Fat: 5.4g, Carbohydrates: 6.6g, Protein: 2.6g

Raspberry Macadamia Crumble

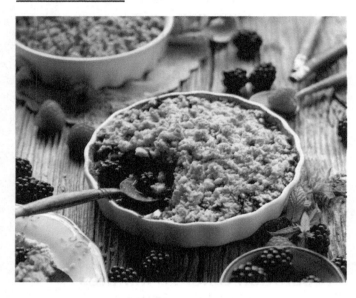

Preparation time: 10 minutes
Cooking time: 25 minutes
Servings: 8

Ingredients:
- 2 cups fresh raspberries
- 2 tablespoons honey
- 2 tablespoons coconut oil
- 1/3 cup rolled oats
- 1/3 cup chopped macadamia nuts
- 1/3 cup shredded coconut
- 1 teaspoon ground cinnamon

Directions:
1. Preheat oven to 350°F (175°C).
2. In a medium bowl, mix together raspberries and honey.
3. In another bowl, mix together coconut oil, rolled oats, chopped macadamia nuts, shredded coconut, and ground cinnamon.
4. Spread the raspberry mixture in an 8-inch baking dish.

5. Sprinkle the oat mixture over the raspberry mixture.
6. Bake for 25 minutes.
7. Let cool before serving.

Nutrition values: Calories: 192, Fat: 12.6g, Carbohydrates: 17.3g, Protein: 3.3g

Baked Apples with Honey and Walnuts

Preparation time: 10 minutes
Cooking time: 25 minutes
Servings: 4

Ingredients:
- 4 large apples, cored and sliced
- 2 tablespoons honey
- 1 teaspoon ground cinnamon
- 2 tablespoons coconut oil
- ¼ cup chopped walnuts

Directions:
1. Preheat oven to 350°F (175°C).
2. Place apples in a large baking dish.
3. Drizzle honey, ground cinnamon, and coconut oil over the apples.
4. Sprinkle walnuts over the apples.
5. Bake for 25 minutes.
6. Let cool before serving.

Nutrition values: Calories: 169, Fat: 8.3g, Carbohydrates: 23.3g, Protein: 1.9g

Lemon Coconut Bars

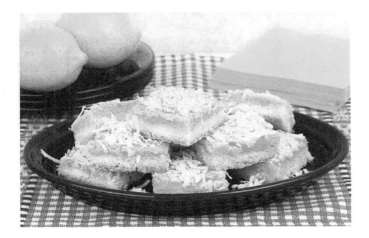

Preparation time: 10 minutes
Cooking time: 30 minutes
Servings: 9

Ingredients:
* 1 cup almond flour
* 2 tablespoons coconut oil
* 2 tablespoons honey
* 2 tablespoons lemon juice
* ½ cup shredded coconut

Directions:
1. Preheat oven to 350°F (175°C).
2. In a medium bowl, mix together almond flour, coconut oil, honey, and lemon juice.
3. Line an 8x8 inch baking dish with parchment paper.
4. Press the dough into the baking dish and spread evenly.
5. Sprinkle shredded coconut over the dough.
6. Bake for 30 minutes.
7. Let cool before serving.

Nutrition values: Calories: 131, Fat: 8.9g, Carbohydrates: 9.8g, Protein: 2.7g

Coconut Mango Popsicles

Preparation time: 15 minutes
Cooking time: 5 minutes

Servings: 8

Ingredients:
* 2 cups diced mango
* 1 cup full-fat coconut milk
* 1/4 cup honey

Directions:
1. Combine the mango, coconut milk, and honey in a blender.
2. Blend until smooth.
3. Pour the mixture into popsicle molds and freeze until solid.

Nutrition values: (per serving)
Calories: 79, Fat: 4g, Carbohydrates: 11g, Protein: 1g

Chocolate Chickpea Blondies

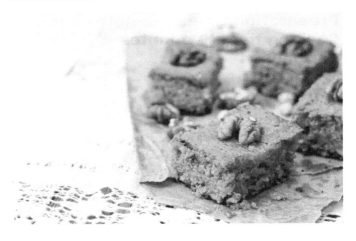

Preparation time: 15 minutes
Cooking time: 30 minutes
Servings: 12

Ingredients:
* 1 1/2 cups cooked chickpeas
* 2/3 cup almond butter
* 1/4 cup maple syrup
* 2 tablespoons cocoa powder
* 1 teaspoon baking powder
* 1/4 teaspoon sea salt
* 1/4 cup mini chocolate chips

Directions:
1. Preheat the oven to 350°F and line an 8x8-inch baking pan with parchment paper.
2. In a food processor, combine the chickpeas, almond butter, maple syrup, cocoa powder, baking powder, and sea salt and blend until smooth.
3. Stir in the chocolate chips.
4. Spread the batter into the prepared baking pan.
5. Bake for 30 minutes.
6. Let cool before slicing and serving.

Nutrition values: (per serving)
Calories: 112, Fat: 6g, Carbohydrates: 11g, Protein: 3g

Chia Seed Pudding with Berries

Preparation time: 5 minutes
Cooking time: 0 minutes
Servings: 4

Ingredients:
- 1 cup unsweetened almond milk
- 1/4 cup chia seeds
- 2 tablespoons honey
- 1 cup fresh berries

Directions:
1. In a medium bowl, whisk together the almond milk, chia seeds, and honey.
2. Refrigerate for at least 4 hours or overnight.
3. Serve topped with fresh berries.

Nutrition values: (per serving)
Calories: 140, Fat: 7g, Carbohydrates: 16g, Protein: 4g

No Bake Tahini Date Balls

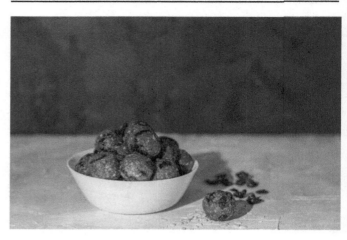

Preparation time: 10 minutes
Cooking time: 0 minutes
Servings: 12

Ingredients:
- 1 cup pitted dates
- 1/2 cup tahini
- 2 tablespoons almond flour
- 1/4 teaspoon ground cinnamon

Directions:
1. In a food processor, combine the dates, tahini, almond flour, and cinnamon and blend until smooth.
2. Roll the mixture into 12 balls.
3. Refrigerate for at least 30 minutes before serving.

Nutrition values: (per serving)
Calories: 87, Fat: 4g, Carbohydrates: 10g, Protein: 2g

BEVERAGE RECIPES

Turmeric Tonic

Preparation time: 5 minutes
Cooking time: 0 minutes
Servings: 1

Ingredients:
- 1 teaspoon of turmeric
- 1 cup of coconut milk
- 1 teaspoon of honey (optional)
- 1 pinch of black pepper
- 1/2 teaspoon of cinnamon

Directions:
1. In a small bowl, mix together the turmeric, coconut milk, honey (optional), black pepper and cinnamon.
2. Pour the mixture into a glass and stir.
3. Drink immediately.

Nutrition Values: Calories: 116; Fat: 11 g; Carbohydrates: 4 g; Protein: 2 g

Beetroot Latte

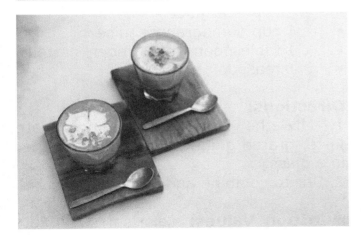

Preparation time: 5 minutes
Cooking time: 5 minutes
Servings: 1

Ingredients:
- 1/2 cup of beetroot juice
- 1/2 cup of coconut milk
- 1/4 teaspoon of cinnamon
- 1 teaspoon of honey (optional)
- Pinch of nutmeg

Directions:
1. In a small saucepan, heat the beetroot juice and coconut milk until it is hot but not boiling.
2. Remove from heat and add the cinnamon, honey (optional) and nutmeg.
3. Pour the mixture into a mug and stir.
4. Enjoy immediately.

Nutrition Values: Calories: 86; Fat: 6 g; Carbohydrates: 6 g; Protein: 1 g

Sweet Potato Smoothie

Preparation time: 5 minutes
Cooking time: 0 minutes
Servings: 1

Ingredients:
- 1 cup of cooked sweet potato, mashed
- 1/2 cup of almond milk
- 1 teaspoon of honey (optional)
- 1/4 teaspoon of cinnamon
- 1/4 teaspoon of nutmeg
- 1/2 banana

Directions:
1. Place all the ingredients in a blender and blend until smooth.
2. Enjoy immediately!

Nutrition Values: Calories: 255; Fat: 5 g; Carbohydrates: 47 g; Protein: 5 g

Blueberry and Kale Juice

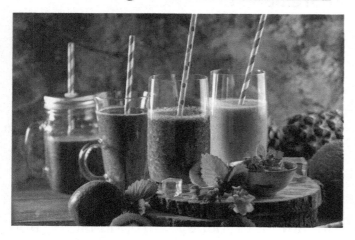

Preparation Time: 5 minutes
Cooking Time: 0 minutes
Servings: 1

Ingredients:
- 1 cup kale
- 1 cup blueberries
- 1 cup coconut water

Directions:
1. Place all ingredients into a blender and blend until smooth.
2. Pour into a glass and enjoy!

Nutrition Values: Calories: 104; Fat: 0.6g; Carbohydrates: 22.3g; Protein: 3.2g

Green Tea and Chia Seed Elixir

Preparation Time: 5 minutes
Cooking Time: 0 minutes
Servings: 1

Ingredients:
- 1 cup brewed green tea
- 1 tablespoon chia seeds
- 1 teaspoon honey

Directions:

1. Brew the green tea and pour into a glass.
2. Add chia seeds and honey and stir to combine.
3. Enjoy!

Nutrition Values: Calories: 67; Fat: 2.6g; Carbohydrates: 10.3g; Protein: 2.3g

Beet and Pomegranate Power Drink

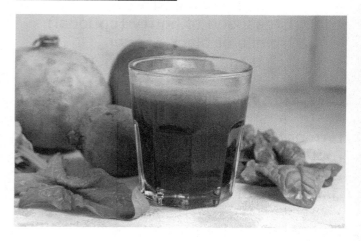

Preparation Time: 5 minutes
Cooking Time: 0 minutes
Servings: 1

Ingredients:
- 1 cup beet juice
- 1 cup pomegranate juice
- 1 tablespoon fresh ginger, grated
- 1 teaspoon honey

Directions:
1. Mix the beet juice, pomegranate juice, grated ginger and honey together in a glass.
2. Stir to combine and enjoy!

Nutrition Values: Calories: 170; Fat: 0.5g; Carbohydrates: 42.3g; Protein: 1.3g

Acai and Avocado Shake

Preparation Time: 10 minutes
Cooking Time: 0 minutes
Servings: 1

Ingredients:
- 1/2 cup frozen acai berries
- 1/2 avocado
- 1 cup unsweetened almond milk
- 1 teaspoon honey
- 1/2 teaspoon ground cinnamon

Directions:
1. Place the acai berries, avocado, almond milk, honey, and cinnamon into a blender.
2. Blend until smooth.
3. Pour into a glass and enjoy!

Nutrition Values: Calories: 323; Fat: 15.3g; Carbohydrates: 35.7g; Protein: 5.7g

Turmeric Latte

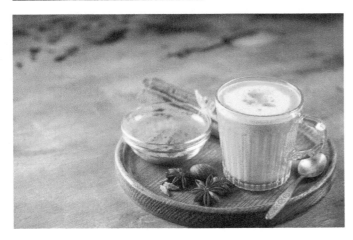

Preparation time: 5 minutes
Cooking time: 5 minutes
Servings: 2

Ingredients:
- 2 cups unsweetened almond milk
- 1 teaspoon ground turmeric
- 1/4 teaspoon ground ginger
- Pinch of ground cinnamon
- 1/4 teaspoon black pepper
- 1 teaspoon pure maple syrup

Directions:
1. Heat the almond milk in a small saucepan over low heat.
2. Whisk in the turmeric, ginger, cinnamon, and black pepper.
3. Bring to a simmer and let cook for 2 minutes.
4. Remove from heat and stir in the maple syrup.
5. Pour into two mugs and enjoy.

Nutrition Values (per serving): Calories: 70; Fat: 3g; Carbohydrates: 6g; Protein: 3g

Pineapple and Cucumber Juice

Preparation time: 10 minutes
Cooking time: None
Servings: 1

Ingredients:
- 1 cup pineapple, peeled and cubed
- 1/2 cup cucumber, peeled and chopped
- 1/2 cup filtered water

Directions:
1. Place all ingredients in a blender and blend until smooth.
2. Strain the juice through a fine mesh strainer and discard the pulp.
3. Pour the juice into a glass and enjoy.

Nutrition Values: Calories: 93; Fat: 0g; Carbohydrates: 24g; Protein: 2g

Ginger and Apple Juice

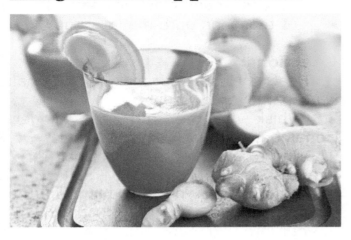

Preparation time: 10 minutes
Cooking time: None
Servings: 1

Ingredients:
- 1 apple, cored and cut into chunks
- 1/4 inch piece of fresh ginger, peeled
- 1 cup filtered water

Directions:
1. Place all ingredients in a blender and blend until smooth.
2. Strain the juice through a fine mesh strainer and discard the pulp.
3. Pour the juice into a glass and enjoy.

Nutrition Values: Calories: 50; Fat: 0g; Carbohydrates: 12g; Protein: 0g

Carrot, Apple and Ginger Juice

Preparation time: 10 minutes
Cooking time: None
Servings: 1

Ingredients:
- 2 carrots, peeled and cut into chunks
- 1 apple, cored and cut into chunks

- 1/4 inch piece of fresh ginger, peeled
- 1 cup filtered water

Directions:
1. Place all ingredients in a blender and blend until smooth.
2. Strain the juice through a fine mesh strainer and discard the pulp.
3. Pour the juice into a glass and enjoy.

Nutrition Values: Calories: 90; Fat: 0g; Carbohydrates: 21g; Protein: 2g

Mango and Turmeric Smoothie

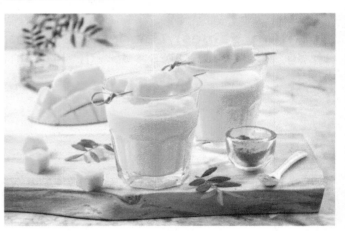

Preparation Time: 10 minutes
Cooking Time: 0 minutes
Servings: 2

Ingredients:
- 1 cup diced mango
- 1/2 teaspoon ground turmeric
- 1/4 teaspoon ground ginger
- 1/4 teaspoon ground cinnamon
- 1 cup almond milk
- 1 tablespoon honey

Directions:
1. Add all ingredients to a blender and blend until smooth. Pour into glasses and serve.

Nutrition Values (per serving): Calories: 111, Fat: 2g, Carbohydrates: 22g, Protein: 2g

Coconut Water and Raspberry Elixir

Preparation Time: 5 minutes
Cooking Time: 0 minutes
Servings: 1

Ingredients:
- 1 cup coconut water
- 1/2 cup frozen raspberries
- 1 teaspoon honey
- 1/4 teaspoon ground turmeric
- 1/8 teaspoon ground ginger

Directions:
1. Add all ingredients to a blender and blend until smooth. Pour into a glass and serve.

Nutrition Values: Calories: 103, Fat: 1g, Carbohydrates: 22g, Protein: 2g

Kale and Spinach Juice

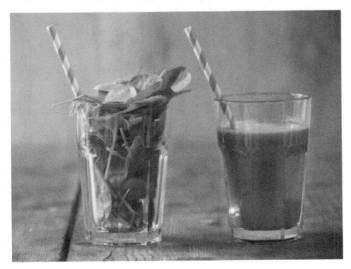

Preparation Time: 5 minutes
Cooking Time: 0 minutes

Servings: 1

Ingredients:
- 2 cups kale leaves
- 2 cups spinach leaves
- 1/2 cup cucumber
- 1/2 cup celery
- 1/2 lemon, juiced
- 1/4 teaspoon ground turmeric
- 1/8 teaspoon ground ginger

Directions:
1. Add all ingredients to a juicer and blend until smooth. Pour into a glass and serve.

Nutrition Values: Calories: 91, Fat: 1g, Carbohydrates: 17g, Protein: 8g

Green Tea and Mint Detox Drink

Preparation Time: 5 minutes
Cooking Time: 0 minutes
Servings: 1

Ingredients:
- 1 teaspoon green tea leaves
- 1/4 cup boiling water
- 1/4 teaspoon honey
- 1/4 teaspoon ground turmeric
- 1/8 teaspoon ground ginger
- 1/2 cup mint leaves

Directions:
1. Add the green tea leaves to a teapot and pour over the boiling water. Let sit for 5 minutes.
2. Strain the tea, add the honey and spices, and stir until dissolved. Add the mint leaves to the mixture and let sit for 5 minutes.
3. Strain and pour into a glass.

Nutrition Values: Calories: 15, Fat: 0g, Carbohydrates: 4g, Protein: 0g

Cucumber and Celery Juice

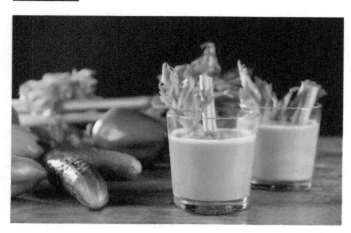

Preparation Time: 10 minutes
Cooking Time: 0 minutes
Servings: 1

Ingredients:
* 2 stalks of celery
* 1 cucumber
* 1/2 cup spinach
* 1/2 cup kale

Directions:
1. Wash and chop the celery and cucumber.
2. Place the celery and cucumber into a juicer and process till all the ingredients have been juiced.
3. Add the spinach and kale and process until all ingredients have been juiced.
4. Serve the juice immediately.

Nutrition Values: Calories: 164; Fat: 1.2 g; Carbohydrates: 38.2 g; Protein: 6.6 g

Beet and Apple Juice

Preparation Time: 10 minutes
Cooking Time: 0 minutes

Servings: 1

Ingredients:
* 1 apple
* 1 beet
* 1/2 cup spinach
* 1/2 cup kale

Directions:
1. Wash and chop the apple and beet.
2. Place the apple and beet into a juicer and process till all the ingredients have been juiced.
3. Add the spinach and kale and process until all ingredients have been juiced.
4. Serve the juice immediately.

Nutrition Values: Calories: 162; Fat: 0.9 g; Carbohydrates: 41.8 g; Protein: 4.2 g

Aloe Vera and Berries Juice

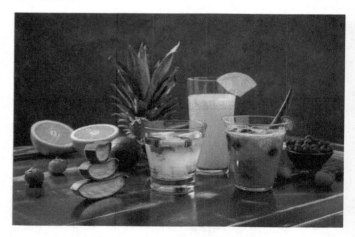

Preparation Time: 10 minutes
Cooking Time: 0 minutes
Servings: 1

Ingredients:
* 1/4 cup aloe vera juice
* 1/2 cup blueberries
* 1/2 cup raspberries
* 1/2 cup blackberries

Directions:
1. Wash and prepare the berries.
2. Place the aloe vera juice and the berries into a juicer and process till all the ingredients have been juiced.
3. Serve the juice immediately.

Nutrition Values: Calories: 118; Fat: 0.8 g; Carbohydrates: 29.5 g; Protein: 1.5 g

Ginger, Lemon and Honey Tea

Preparation Time: 10 minutes
Cooking Time: 5 minutes
Servings: 1

Ingredients:

- 1 cup water
- 1/2 teaspoon grated ginger
- 1 teaspoon honey
- 1 teaspoon lemon juice

Directions:
1. Bring the water to a boil in a small saucepan.
2. Add in the grated ginger and reduce the heat to low.
3. Simmer for 5 minutes.
4. Remove from heat and add the honey and lemon juice.
5. Stir to combine.
6. Strain the tea into a mug and serve.

Nutrition Values: Calories: 58; Fat: 0.1 g; Carbohydrates: 15.2 g; Protein: 0.3 g

28-DAY MEAL PLAN

DAY	BREAKFAST	LUNCH	DINNER	DESSERTS
1	Oats with strawberries	Chicken with sweet potato	Quinoa Bowl	Apple Crumble with toasted coconut
2	Scrambled egg and vegetable wrap	Grilled Salmon with dill	Stuffed Peppers	Banana date Walnut Bars
3	Yogurt Parfait with fruit	Avocado toast	Grilled chicken burgers	Lemon coconut bars
4	Banana Oat Smoothie bowl	Coconut curry chicken	Spinach artichoke dip	Raspberry macadamia crumble
5	Omelet with spinach, mushrooms...	Grilled sardines	Quinoa salad	Lemon coconut bars
6	Acai bowl with hemp seeds	Slow cooker chicken and rice soup	Portobello burgers	Cocoa almond bites
7	Kale, tomato and avocado scramble egg	Carrot sticks with hummus	Cajun-style red snapper	No bake tahini date balls
8	Gluten free fruit & nut granola	Vegetable Lasagna	Broiled cod with mango	Strawberry rhubarb crumble
9	Avocado toast with poached egg	Tuna salad on whole wheat crackers	Grilled lamb chops with mango	Spiced pear galette
10	Chia seed pudding with coconut...	Tomato basil frittata	Baked tilapia with olives & tomato	Chocolate chickpea blondies
11	Sweet potato hash with	Trail mix	Chicken thighs with apples...	Zucchini cake with lemon

			glaze
12	Red lentil and zucchini fritters	Poached cod with lemon - capper sauce	Falafel platter	Apple with cinnamon and maple syrup
13	Burrito with sweet potato & beans	Pan – fried salmon with spinach...	Vegetarian chili	Almond butter brownies
14	Buckwheat porridge with apple...	Chicken breasts with mushrooms...	Grilled vegetable skewers	Coconut flour carrot cake
15	Turmeric latte with coconut milk	Roasted ratatouille	Mahi-mahi with pineapple salsa	Coconut mango popsicles
16	Coconut quinoa porridge	Grilled barramundi with tomato...	Eggplant parmesan	Sweet potato brownies
17	Almond flour pancakes with banana...	Cucumber slices with cheese	Salmon and asparagus	Blueberry almond flour muffins
18	Smoked salmon and frittata	Backed lemon garlic chicken	Pasta salad	Chocolate avocado pudding
19	Quinoa breakfast	Pork tenderloin & vegetables	Mahi-mahi with coconut – lime sauce	Banana oat blondies
20	Poached egg, asparagus & tomato	Sirloin steak with avocado salsa	Spinach artichoke dip	Apples with honey & walnuts
21	Oats with strawberries	Pulled chicken with sweet potatoes	Stuffed peppers	Apple crumble with coconut
22	Avocado toast with poached egg	Mackerel with lemon-garlic butter	Quinoa bowl	Banana date walnut bars
23	Scrambled egg and vegetable	Bison burger with avocado	Veggie wraps	Strawberry rhubarb

	wrap			crumble
24	Chia seed pudding with coconut, milk, and berries	Grilled halibut with mango salsa	Pan-fried salmon with spinach and tomatoes	No bake tahini date balls
25	Banana oat smoothie bowl	Greek yogurt	Grilled teriyaki chicken	Zucchini cake with lemon glaze
26	Acai bowl with hemp seeds	Broiled cod with mango salsa	Falafel platter	Coconut flower carrot cake
27	Smoked salmon and spinach frittata	Chicken cacciatore	Kale chips	Baked apples with cinnamon and maple syrup
28	Buckwheat porridge with apple and cinnamon	Coconut curry chicken	Mediterranean pasta salad	Spiced pear galette

WEEKLY SHOPPING LIST

VEGETABLES
- Peppers
- Spinach
- Quinoa
- Mushrooms
- Basil
- Tomato
- Eggplant
- Potato
- Asparagus
- Zucchini
- Lentil
- Capper
- Carrot
- Cauliflower

FRUITS
- Apple
- Banana
- Avocado
- Coconut
- Pear
- Mango
- Strawberries
- Blueberry
- Lemon

DAIRY
- Cheese
- Coconut milk
- Milk
- Butter
- Yogurt
- Parmesan

CONDIMENTS, HERBS & SPICES
- Garlic
- Onion
- Chili
- Rosemary
- Cinnamon
- Ginger
- Mint
- Cumin

MEAT
- Poultry
- Pork
- Lamb
- Beef
- Turkey

FISH & SEAFOOD
- Salmon
- Tilapia
- Mahi-mahi
- Cod

OTHER
- Egg
- Pasta
- Beans
- Quinos
- Chocolate

Made in the USA
Coppell, TX
22 April 2023

15941761R00044